Author of "*God's Weigh to Your Ideal Body Weight*" &
"*The Cult of Calvinism*"
<u>**Prayer, Amazon Review, & Ministry Donations appreciated**</u>
17223 Mesa Springs Court, Houston, TX 77095
www.godsweighministry.com
michaelscottlowery@yahoo.com
832-331-6826

GOD'S WEIGH
TO YOUR
IDEAL BODY WEIGHT

YOUR BODY
SHOULD
GLORIFY GOD

MICHAEL SCOTT LOWERY

Founder of
God's Weigh Ministry
http://www.godsweighministry.com/

WESTBOW
P R E S S
A DIVISION OF THOMAS NELSON

WestBow Press books may be ordered through booksellers or by contacting:

WestBow Press
A Division of Thomas Nelson
1663 Liberty Drive
Bloomington, IN 47403
www.westbowpress.com
1-(866) 928-1240

ISBN: 978-1-4497-8657-1 (sc)
ISBN: 978-1-4497-8659-5 (hc)
ISBN: 978-1-4497-8658-8 (e)
Library of Congress Control Number: 2013903355

Printed in the United States of America
WestBow Press rev. date: 3/13/2013

Table of Contents

Preface

Year after year the number one New Year's resolution is weight loss. Yet, year after year we continue to lose the battle of the bulge in ever-increasing degrees. I think it could be argued that the worship of the body-beautiful has continued to increase year after year as well. We often consider this to be a tragedy of health, which it certainly is. But isn't this also an incredible emotional tragedy? While our desire to look good increases, our health and looks are decreasing even quicker.

The poor physical condition of the people in this country, and even around the world in recent decades, is more dramatic and epic a catastrophe as presented by any plague in the Bible. With the exception of the world flood, no plague in Scripture was more damaging and on a more global scale than the degeneration we have seen in the health and body weight of people around the world. Something must be wrong.

How can this be? There is a new diet plan or exercise program out on the market even before the previous diet plan or exercise program has fizzled out. But despite the promises made, none provide sustainable success. Mankind has done its best to resolve the health and body weight issues of the people in this country and around the world. The world has responded optimistically to these man-made solutions with the expenditure of billions of dollars each year on gym memberships, diet and exercise programs, the latest fitness equipment, the most wiz-bang kitchen appliances imaginable, and nutritional supplements, but to no avail.

Mankind has even decided that since we can't seem to figure out how to improve our health and body weight, we should now come up with some pop-psychology that will help us to learn to accept ourselves just the way we are. Is the problem not that we are overweight after all, but that we simply lack self-esteem and have a poor body image? Is big beautiful? That doesn't sound right.

The Church can't argue, or hasn't argued, that this problem is caused by a lack of Godly wisdom and power. The Church can't argue this because the Church is just as tired, sick, and overweight as the rest of the world. Should this be the case? Or should the Church have access to God's wisdom concerning this matter, wisdom that the world could never have known or discerned?

If the Church should be able to look to God for wisdom to overcome this issue, then why has it not? The Church contends that God has provided us with the wisdom and power to live a successful life, but at least relative to health and body weight, that has not been proven to be true. Has God failed us in this area? Did He fail to show us a better way? Should the Church be looking to the world for the answer? Up until now that has certainly been the case. Shouldn't the world be looking to the Church for answers and solutions to life's challenges?

We obviously believe that our body weight is of serious importance. It wouldn't be number one on the New Year's resolution list if it wasn't. Is it possible that God would have failed to provide instruction regarding an area that is that important to us? Could God have forgotten to equip us to be successful in achieving good health, and in reaching and maintaining our ideal body weight? I really would have thought that God cared more about His people than that.

Maybe God has provided His people with the wisdom and power to live successfully with regard to health and body weight. If so, how would the Church have missed His instructions? With the constant study of the Bible, by millions of scholars and laymen alike, on a daily basis, with such a huge problem looming above our heads, it doesn't seem possible that we would have overlooked such incredible insights.

Is Satan to blame? Satan is always the thief that comes to kill, steal, and destroy. Is this his handiwork? It certainly makes sense that Satan would want to keep God's best from us. But if we are so concerned about our health and body weight, how could he have deceived us into ignoring God's wisdom regarding the matter?

Could it be that the Church has willingly ignored God's instructions, maybe because they have been deemed too difficult? But in order to do this, wouldn't the Church have to misinterpret God's Word, deny that such wisdom existed, and/or deny that it applied to us today? If this wisdom is the solution we are looking for, why would it not apply to us today? If it doesn't apply then maybe God isn't concerned about our health and body weight after all. So why did He go to all the trouble of including His instructions regarding diet and health in the Bible? It all just doesn't make sense. Until now...

Introduction

If you are struggling with excess body weight then you have come to the right place. *God's Weigh to Your Ideal Body Weight* is the <u>Biblical</u> path to reaching your ideal body weight. If you are overweight you will lose fat. If you are underweight, whether from the effects of anorexia, bulimia, or poor health, you will gain muscle and a healthy level of fat. And in all cases, you will learn how to achieve spiritual, emotional, and physical health through Godly wisdom.

God has a message for you today. He wants you to reach your ideal body weight. And He wants to tell you how to achieve it. God has given you His Word, the Bible, to do just that. *God's Weigh to Your Ideal Body Weight* uncovers the plan for health and weight loss as prescribed by the Creator of your body. I use the word 'uncovers' not because God has tried to hide it from you but because most people don't seem to know that God's wisdom concerning diet and weight loss is in the Bible to begin with.

As a Believer, it is your birthright to live out your life at your ideal body weight. This is part of God's will for your life. God has provided everything you need to know to get there in the Bible. But just as Esau, we have sold that birthright to satisfy our fleshly lusts. It's time to take it back!

God knows that living at your ideal body weight is an important part of living the abundant life that you desire, the abundant life that He desires for you. There is no point allowing anyone to convince you that living at 25, 50, 75, 100+ pounds overweight is an abundant way to live.

God is not asking you to determine a way to mentally and emotionally accept your excess body weight and poor vitality. God is not asking you to learn to accept failure in your Christian walk. God wants to provide you with the wisdom and power necessary for successful living, to include the success of living your life at your ideal body weight.

The Bible is the greatest health and weight loss book ever written. For example, in only 10 words, God reveals what you are to eat, how much you are to eat, when you are to eat, and why you are to eat (dietary holiness). And He goes on to tell you what it takes to become spiritually conditioned to the point of obedience to His dietary directives in route to your ideal body weight.

As harsh as it may sound, God is not glorified when His people are overweight. We are called to glorify God in our bodies, to be a witness to the world, to be a light that shines on a hill, and to live above all the nations. The Church is called to be a beacon of hope, an example of successful living, and a testimony to the wisdom and power of God in our lives. An overweight Church fails to accomplish this God-ordained calling to its fullest potential.

The Church should be the healthiest demographic on the planet. We have the wisdom and power of God through the Bible and the Holy Spirit to equip us, to furnish us, unto all good works. The world would be so impressed with our success in the area of reaching and maintaining our ideal body weights alone that they would be beating down our church doors to find out what we were doing differently, why we were doing it differently, and Who told us to do it differently; thereby offering one of the greatest evangelical opportunities the Church has ever known!

There is such a thing as dietary holiness; God's standard for holy living concerning our dietary practices. And there is such a thing as dietary deception, which is the work of Satan, in conjunction with the cooperation of our fleshly natures, to deny that God has a call upon our lives to walk holy in the area of diet. The Church has misinterpreted, even modified, Scripture to justify their acceptance of dietary deception and its negative fruit in our lives.

Through dietary deception God's people have become tired, sick, overweight, and are living a fraction of the years God intended. Consider lifespan. God says that we should live 120 years in Genesis 6:3. He then goes on to say in Psalm 90:7-12 that a people living in sin will only live 70 to 80 years, exactly how long we are living today. This should not be. God tells us that we will know evil by its evil fruit. Wisdom is screaming in the streets, to the Church and to you.

Through spiritual conditioning and God's dietary directives you will reach and maintain your ideal body weight. It's your birthright, achievable through dietary holiness. Don't allow Satan to steal your birthright any longer through dietary deception.

You will be able to reach your ideal body weight as you begin to see and apply God's plan for your diet and health. And equally important, you will be able to reach your ideal body weight as you see the deceptions of Satan and mankind regarding health and weight loss exposed.

Over the course of reading this book you will learn terms that may be unfamiliar to you. These terms will include spiritual conditioning, dietary disclaimer, dietary holiness, dietary deception, secret sin, the legalism lie, dietary reformation, and the Biblical Doctrine of Physical Health to name a few. These are all terms I have developed and/or found in Scripture to describe the Biblical principles that will help you reach your ideal body weight.

I am very excited for you. You are about to learn what very few people know. You are about to learn what God, the Creator of your body, has to say about diet and health. And through God's wisdom and power concerning diet and health you are about to start your journey towards your ideal body weight.

I know of your struggles and the pain you have experienced. I know of the foolish ideas of man that have only made things worse for you, that have led to poor health and an overweight body. Satan wants you to continue to suffer. He is the ultimate enemy to your objective of reaching your ideal body weight. I want to help you take back the ground he has stolen in your life through dietary deception.

What I refer to as the Biblical Doctrine of Physical Health includes diet, rest, fasting, healing, forgiveness, loving others, and a whole lot more. But for the purposes of this book, helping you reach your ideal body weight, diet will be our primary focus. Diet is where the majority of reformation is needed in your life to enable you to reach your ideal body weight.

My intent is not to try to provide you with a method or formula for determining your specific ideal body weight. For two women of the same height, due to differences in skeletal structure and tendencies toward varying levels of musculature, the ideal body weight for one may be 120 pounds while the ideal body weight for the other may be 135 pounds. So you will not be seeing any height-weight charts in this book. God knows what your ideal body weight should be, and you will know it when you get there.

The pace at which you travel towards your ideal body weight will depend on how unhealthy your body is initially; that is, your level of physical conditioning. And the pace at which you can successfully live a life that creates a healthy body will depend upon how out of shape you are spiritually, your level of spiritual conditioning.

Although body weight might be largely controllable via the Biblical wisdom found in this book regarding diet, your overall health can be ruined as quickly by unforgiveness and bitterness, for example, as by a regular diet of soda, candy, tobacco, and alcohol. It is the whole picture of God's plan and purpose for your life that you must pursue, even as you dig deeper into a topic-specific area like diet and health.

Do you want to pass down a heritage of spiritual, emotional, and physical weakness to your children and grandchildren? Do you want them to suffer as you have? Are you ready for the truth, no matter what the cost, in order to bless their futures as well as yours?

You have seen that the Christian community is arguably the most tired, sick, and overweight demographic on the planet. Something must be wrong. How could the proper application of God's grace and mercy, and all of the truths of God's Word, possibly lead to this result?

God tells us that we will know evil by its evil fruit. An overweight body is evil fruit. It is just that simple. An overweight body is the result of living in defiance to God's Word regarding diet and health. A body at its ideal weight is righteous fruit, the result of living in obedience to God's Word.

I am hopeful for you. My hope is not a wish. My hope for you is founded in the promises, wisdom, and power of God's Word. I know that the same promises, wisdom, and power that have set me free from addiction to food, unhealthy eating, poor health, and excess weight will do the same for you.

Have you had enough? Are you ready for the truth, the whole truth, and nothing but the truth? Are you ready for a dietary reformation in your own life and in the Church? That is what this book is all about. If so, then you are ready to take back the birthright of living out your life at your ideal body weight.

As you read through this book, trying to discern the truth of Scripture regarding diet and health, please apply the following acid test to differentiate between what is true and what is false.

1) Are the principles found in this book balanced with respect to God's love, God's holiness, and God's sovereignty? I think you will find that dietary holiness strikes the perfect balance.

2) When deciding between two opposite Biblical views, break the tie by determining which view gives God the most glory. I think you will find that dietary holiness, as opposed to dietary deception, will give God the most glory.

3) The Bible says we will know evil by its evil fruit. Determine which

view leads towards righteous fruit and which view leads towards evil fruit. I think you will find that dietary holiness produces righteous fruit and dietary deception produces evil fruit.

God is calling for dietary holiness in your life and in the Church. God wants you to be at your ideal body weight. He wants this for every Believer.

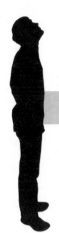
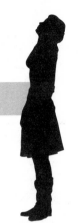

Chapter 1

The Bible is the Greatest Health & Weight Loss Book Ever Written

I have spent over 30 years in the study of diet and health; the first 13 years totally devoted to worldly wisdom on the subject, and the next 17 years devoted primarily to God's Word. I have sought God regarding the issue of diet and health through Bible study, prayer, the study of countless books and articles regarding health, my own trial and error, and the process of spiritual growth.

With the exception of some interesting scientific insights into how the body works, all of the non-Biblical study I have performed over those many years has been a waste of time, at the very least, unnecessary. Even more than that, the non-Biblical study actually worked to harm me and keep me from God's diet and health plan. It kept me from my ideal body weight. It was only complete adherence and reliance on God's Word that enabled me to reach my ideal body weight.

Although you will certainly benefit from my efforts through this book, you should always seek God directly for wisdom regarding all matters. God's wisdom is not reserved for a select few, but to those who will diligently seek Him.

"If any of you lacks wisdom, let him ask of God, who gives to all liberally and without reproach, and it will be given to him." (James 1:5, NKJV, BibleGateway.com)

Even the most well-intentioned person can lead you down the road to failure if their message is not Biblically sound. There is an important Christian life principle in this. Never inherit your theology from man! It will be through God's Word, not man's opinion, that you determine whether or not you are living in sin relative to diet and health, and what it means to walk in righteousness.

"Thy word have I hid in mine heart, that I might not sin against thee." (Psalm 119:11, KJV)

I see so much theological error in the Christian community that has occurred simply because many Christians will hold to a certain Biblical view on a subject because their grandfather held to that view, their pastor held to that view, their favorite TV evangelist held to that view, or the most popular person at church held to that view. But it was not because they had sought God and His Word directly for wisdom regarding that subject. This is a dangerous practice.

This book is God's Weigh, not man's way, to your ideal body weight. God tells us that the wisdom of man will only get us into more trouble than that with which we started. At best, man's way can only put a temporary bandage on the symptoms of a much greater problem, even working to help ensure you never reach your goals in most cases. It is only God and His wisdom that can lead you to true, complete success in any area of your life, reaching your ideal body weight included.

"Trust in the LORD with all your heart, and lean not on your own understanding. In all your ways acknowledge Him, and He shall direct your paths. Do not be wise in your own eyes. Fear the LORD and depart from evil. It will be health to your flesh and strength to your bones." (Proverbs 3:5-8, NKJV, BibleGateway.com)

Although this passage has application to every area of your life, it makes a direct reference to achieving physical health in verse 8. 'Departing from evil' and walking in obedience to God's Word is the way to 'health to your flesh,' to 'strength to your bones,' and to your ideal body weight.

Even before buying this book, you may have already discovered (strongly considered) that God might care about your body weight and health. You are way ahead of most if you have come to that realization. But you may have then moved on to other sources to determine a way to achieve those things in your life.

Please get this. If God is concerned about a particular matter in our lives, He will also be the source of how to achieve success regarding that matter. This is an important life principle that will serve you well in reaching your ideal body weight, and in every other area of your life. This is true for the topics of salvation, marriage, parenting, work, finances, serving others, relationships, prophecy, and yes, diet and health.

Have we really thought that God failed to provide us with instructions regarding diet and health? We certainly act like God has nothing for us, to help us reach our ideal body weight. Maybe it is more that we have decided we don't want what God has for us. We may be unwilling to 'go there,' hoping mankind will come up with a more convenient plan than what God might have to offer.

Have we refused to turn to God regarding weight loss because we unconsciously believe it is a fleshly desire, not wanting His light shed upon some unrighteous motivation? Although I believe that is part of the reason, I think that it is also that most assume God doesn't care about such things. I think most of us have assumed that concern over our body weight and health is not a spiritual matter. I think most of us have failed to realize that our concern over our body weight may be the work of the Holy Spirit in our lives. The Holy Spirit may be working to lead us to God and to show us the error in our lives that has led to an undesired body weight.

Have we refused to turn to God regarding weight loss because we simply didn't know He spoke to such things? He speaks to every other major facet of our lives. Did He forget to thoroughly address an area of our lives that takes up an incredible amount of our time and thought, second maybe only to sleep and work?

Let me assure you right now. God does care about your body weight. Your concern over your body weight is the working of the Holy Spirit in your life to lead you to God's truth and solution. The Bible is full of God's directives concerning diet and health. The Bible is the greatest health and weight loss book ever written. You will see that in the pages ahead.

I see it so often in the Christian community, that we will decide God wants certain things to happen in this world – in our lives – in our church, and we may be exactly right. But then we leave Him on the shelf and seek after man's wisdom as to how to achieve it. For example, on occasion a church leader will decide that health should be promoted in their church as part of a Godly life-style, a good revelation. But then this church leader will embrace and apply a fitness program produced and promoted by someone who is not a Christian, by someone who has certainly never sought God regarding fitness and who makes no reference to God whatsoever. The church leader wrongly assumes that God has nothing to say on the matter.

The Church doesn't need to go to the world for wisdom, the topic of diet and health included. That is a terrible thing, but the Church does it all the time. The world should be beating down the Church's door demanding to know why we are healthier than they, why we are living longer than they, and why we are not overweight like every other demographic. We are the ones with God's wisdom and power available to us, not them.

If God's ways are higher than man's ways then we had better make sure that whatever instruction we are seeking and receiving comes from God. If we want the best in our lives we had better go to the right source for the ultimate in wisdom and power. Concerning diet, health, and reaching your ideal body weight, does it not make sense that you seek out the Creator of your body first?

"For my thoughts are not your thoughts, neither are your ways my ways, saith the Lord. For as the heavens are higher than the earth, so are my ways higher than your ways, and my thoughts than your thoughts." (Isaiah 55:8-9, KJV)

It is important that you get your priorities straight and do things in the proper order. As tempting as it may be, you must never allow any book, even one about the Bible, including this one, to take precedence over your time in direct Bible study and prayer. I would suggest you commit a minimum of 30 minutes each day to direct Bible study and prayer before moving on to a book someone has written about the Bible.

I have noticed that many Christians today are open and even anxious to participate in book studies of books written about the Bible, while spending much less time directly in God's Word. I have seen this tendency increasing with each passing year, putting the Christian individual, and the Church overall, at risk in several ways.

One, we can become more open to inheriting incorrect theologies from man. Two, there is something about the spiritual power that is derived from direct Bible study that can be found no other way. Three, topic-specific books, if the only thing being read, will not provide a more whole, balanced picture of God's plan and purpose for our lives as we dig deeply into only the one topic addressed in a particular book. And four, the study of a book about the Bible can lend itself to too much time spent on the technical aspects (or the do's and don'ts) that are promoted as keys to success in a particular area, and not enough time emphasizing the spiritual conditioning that must form the foundation for success in any topic-specific area.

Don't ever be deceived into believing that God doesn't speak to such practical issues as diet and health in the Bible. You could throw away every diet and health book ever written, including this one (although I might help save you some time and energy), and you would do extremely well with the Bible alone. The Bible is the greatest health and weight loss book ever written!!!

"All scripture is given by inspiration of God, and is profitable for doctrine, for reproof, for correction, for instruction in righteousness: that the man of God may be perfect, thoroughly furnished unto all good works." (II Timothy 3:16, KJV)

If you are overweight and unhealthy, can you say 'I am thoroughly furnished unto all good works?' Of course not. You may not even feel like getting off the couch due to fatigue and depression about your physical condition, much less feeling up to good works.

Out of the necessity to make money to live on, you may be forcing your way through your work days, requiring a level of determination and suffering that is actually quite remarkable in its own right. I want you to see that you are not overweight because you are lazy and apathetic, quite the contrary.

I can sympathize with this type of existence in my own life. I know what it means to be 40 pounds over my ideal body weight, living in a chronic state of fatigue. I also know what it means to apply God's wisdom concerning diet, lose those 40 pounds, and have an endless supply of energy.

You are overweight because you are deficient in seeking out and operating by God's wisdom. You may actually be one of the most determined and well-meaning people on the planet. But you see, if Satan can sidetrack you through a life lived by ungodly principles, even if your heart is in the right place, he can make hidden even the greatest qualities with which God has endowed you.

"For You formed my inward parts. You covered me in my mother's womb. I will praise You for I am fearfully and wonderfully made. Marvelous are Your works. And that my soul knows very well." (Psalm 139:13-14, NKJV, BibleGateway.com)

So get the belief that you are overweight because you are 'lazy' or a 'lesser person than those thin folks' out of your mind right now. You wouldn't have bought this book if that was true. Satan wants you to believe that you are overweight because you are a weak person. It is important in life that you learn to recognize the voice of Satan that works its way into your thinking.

God doesn't make junk. You are anything but that. God says so. It is Satan who has deceived you into believing otherwise. It is Satan who is working to keep you from the wisdom of God's Word that can set you free. It is Satan who has deceived you into believing that desiring to be at your ideal body weight is some evil, shallow wish. Satan certainly doesn't want you to know that it is God's will for your life to reach your ideal body weight and that it is your birthright as a Believer.

If you are overweight it simply means that you have gone down a path that is void of Godly wisdom and power regarding diet and health. Like most, you may not even be aware that God cares about your body weight and the struggles you have had regarding it. And like most, you certainly have not been made aware that God has spoken very powerfully and directly to the matters of diet and health in the Bible. You have missed out on receiving the kind of information/wisdom and encouragement you have needed and been looking for all along. That is all about to change.

Not only should you be diligent to seek God's wisdom directly through Bible study and prayer, but you must be extremely wary of what mankind offers in the way of solutions to life's challenges. Nobody needs to tell you that mankind has done all it can to develop a plan for everyone to reach their ideal body weight, the result being a dismal failure.

"*There is a way which seemeth right unto a man, but the end thereof are the ways of death.*" (Proverbs 14:12, KJV)

No matter how fancy the program, how sparkly the equipment, or how charismatic the founder, these programs keep failing time after time, attempt after attempt. Isn't it time that you give God a shot at helping you reach your ideal body weight? Isn't it time you looked to the Bible, the greatest health and weight loss book ever written?

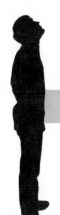

Chapter 2

Dietary Directives, Dietary Holiness, Dietary Deception, & The Legalism Lie

I have and will continue to toss around the terms dietary directives, dietary holiness, and dietary deception throughout the book, as well as address the topic of legalism. I will address each briefly in the order listed here. Although I address these terms in much greater depth and detail later in the book, I would encourage you to read this book in the order the chapters have been presented.

The entirety of what is fully involved in these Biblical principles/terms is quite extensive and spiritually challenging (very deep stuff), necessitating that you grow in the wisdom and power of God's Word as you study through the book before addressing these terms in a more concentrated and comprehensive manner later on.

When I mention dietary directives I am not talking about Scott's dietary directives. I am referring to God's dietary directives. The term dietary directive brings with it an understanding that God's dietary plan is not a suggestion to be considered, but rather a commandment to be obeyed. This is not to say that obedience to God's Word concerning diet is a requirement for salvation. That would be legalism. But what this term does mean is that God has a standard for our dietary practices and He expects us to walk in obedience to His Word regarding it.

The term dietary holiness refers to the fact that obedience to God's dietary directives is a component of Godly, righteous living; a part of holy living. Putting the two words together, dietary and holiness, make this principle concise and clear.

In contrast to dietary holiness, there is dietary deception. Dietary deception, in a nutshell, is the work of Satan in the Church to keep Believers from understanding the principles of dietary directives, dietary holiness, and everything and anything to do with God's Word concerning diet and health. Further, dietary deception includes misconceptions and misinterpretations of Scripture used in an effort by Satan, in cooperation with the willingness of our fleshly lusts and natures, to cause Believers to deny that such principles are even Biblical and/or applicable.

The remainder of this book will work to demonstrate the Biblical accuracy and applicability of dietary directives, dietary holiness, and dietary deception to your life and to your journey to reach your ideal body weight.

The legalism lie is an essential component of dietary deception; possibly the number one tool of the enemy to keep God's people from dietary holiness and their ideal body weights. Although 'legalism' is not a word that appears in the Bible, it has been coined to address a particular Biblical principle.

The problem has been that the Church either doesn't define this term correctly and/or applies it to something that doesn't fit the correct definition. Nowhere is this more evident than with respect to dietary holiness.

The act of legalism occurs when someone contends that something other than faith is required for eternal salvation. For example, if I said that God doesn't want you to lie, is that legalism? No. It would only have been legalism if I said that anyone who lies cannot be saved; that honesty is a requirement for earning and maintaining your eternal salvation.

What if I said God wants every Believer to wear a red shirt every day? Would that be legalism? Many would say yes, but it is not. It may or may not be true that God wants every Believer to wear a red shirt every day. That isn't the issue. You see, I did not say that wearing a red shirt every day was a requirement for earning and maintaining your eternal salvation. Only then would I have been both wrong <u>and</u> legalistic.

As Believers, we are called to live holy lives before God. But our eternal salvation is not dependent upon our obedience to God with regard to diet and health. To say otherwise would be legalism. A component of holy living is dietary holiness, or adherence to God's dietary directives. Dietary holiness is not a requirement for eternal salvation; therefore, the claim that Believers are called to a life of dietary holiness cannot be labeled legalism.

No one is arguing that abiding by God's dietary directives is a requirement for salvation. But I hope this book proves to you that God's dietary directives are a component of holy living.

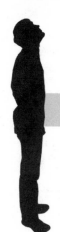

Chapter 3

Diet & Body Weight in Perspective

Walking in obedience to God's Word concerning your dietary practices (dietary holiness) will be essential to achieving health and reaching your ideal body weight. That being said, there are other factors, some you can control and some that you cannot control, that affect your overall health. Just because you reach your ideal body weight does not mean that you can be guaranteed to be 100% perfectly healthy, although the likelihood increases exponentially.

What I refer to as the Biblical Doctrine of Physical Health is made up of more than just God's dietary directives. The Biblical Doctrine of Physical Health includes diet, rest, fasting, and healing, for example. And it also includes forgiveness, purposeful living, and other areas of Christian living that we do not tend to equate with physical health, but do in fact affect it. A life lived in unforgiveness and bitterness can destroy your health as quickly as a steady diet of alcohol, tobacco, and donuts. For the most part, these non-diet topics will be beyond the scope of this book, although I will make several points along the way regarding how some of these can work to affect your body weight.

There are also factors beyond your control, at least in the immediate, which work to negatively affect your overall health. These factors can include general pollution in the environment, possible long-term negative effects from some inoculations, and various diseases that can be contracted from the world around us that may or may not be healed through dietary holiness alone.

Less easily controllable factors can also include the quality of the food we have available to us, even God-approved foods (the only kind that should be called food to begin with), because of the manner in which mankind has worked to make them available to us. These might include foods brought to maximum production through the use of chemicals and pesticides, grain-fed verses grass-fed animal and dairy products, growth hormones used to raise animals for consumption, and maybe even foods grown and harvested out of season. Addressing these factors is beyond the scope of this book.

But whether controllable or not in the immediate term, these factors are things the Christian community needs to take seriously. Relative to those factors you can control, you should begin seeking God and taking steps to improve in those areas. Relative to those factors you cannot control in the immediate, there is still a need for you and the Christian community to be part of the solution to these problems in our society.

For the purpose and scope of this book, as we are addressing God's dietary plan for you, we will be talking primarily about your basic dietary choices. The purpose of this book is not to get into grass-fed verse grain-fed beef, for example. I am not saying this is not an important issue, but at this stage in your journey towards dietary holiness, getting your basic dietary choices down will be where you need to start.

Let me define 'basic dietary choices' for you. A basic dietary choice would be the basic choice between consuming an orange and a donut, for example. This choice would not include dietary health factors such as the soil quality within which the food was grown, whether the food was organically grown or subjected to various chemical fertilizers and pesticides, whether or not the food has been pasteurized and/or homogenized, or if growth hormones and antibiotics were used, for example. The issue at hand is determining which item is God-approved for your consumption and how to develop the spiritual strength to make the right choice.

Many of you have worked to address those 'other' concerns in your life and in your communities. This is certainly an important part of dietary reformation. However, for the Church to worry about these 'other' dietary health factors, before learning to control its basic dietary choices, may not be the best investment of our time and energies at this stage.

If you are at a place where you are still choosing a donut over an orange, it may not be all that important to worry about, and spend time with pursuing, organic foods. Your best investment in time will be in gaining the spiritual strength to control your basic dietary choices. What is better, an organic donut or a non-organic orange? You need to get your basic dietary choices down first.

If I had to put a very conservative number to it, I would contend that our basic dietary choices constitute <u>at least</u> one-third of the overall influence on health of the various health factors included in the Biblical Doctrine of Physical Health, let's say 35% for discussion's sake.

In other words, over 35% of our health problems come about simply because we chose a donut over an orange, because we chose coke over water, because we choose refined sugar over honey, or because we simply overeat, for example. 35% of the difference between how long God says we should live and how long we are actually living should be taken back, which comes out to an extra 15 years above the average 75-year life span, or 90 years (120 less 75 all multiplied by 35%). We will discuss lifespan later.

More importantly, of all the health factors involved, I believe that the bulk of our spiritual issues associated with diet and other health factors can be found lurking in the area of our basic dietary choices. If we will grow spiritually in the wisdom and application of God's Word to our basic dietary choices, all of the other health factors can then begin to fall into place over time.

Your inability to control your basic dietary choices brings into play spiritual issues equal or greater in magnitude and significance to most Biblical topics. Lust, idol worship, greed, pride, Biblical misinterpretation, the unwillingness to search the Scriptures for truth, improper parenting, and general disobedience are some of the spiritual issues involved in just your basic dietary choices. God's dietary directives are no small matter.

It really doesn't matter whether our basic dietary choices are 100%, 50%, or only 25% of the problem, or solution, as the case may be. God has given us His commands concerning diet, and they are to be followed. It is not up to us to determine whether we should be motivated to obey or not based on the consequences or impact determined. For what it's worth, I think the right number is closer to 50-60%.

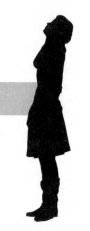

Chapter 4

Exercise is Not Necessary to Reach Your Ideal Body Weight

Despite what the show The Biggest Loser might communicate, reaching your ideal body weight does not require an exercise program, or in their case, excessive exercise. You could be bed-ridden and still reach your ideal body weight. And for me, it would be a toss-up between wanting to lose the excess weight 'fast and furious' their way and not wanting a bunch of loose skin on my body.

The Biggest Loser method is not God's Weigh. God's Weigh to your ideal body weight will allow your body to rebalance its hormones in a gradual and healthy manner, greatly reducing or eliminating the incidence of loose skin. Also, The Biggest Loser method would have you counting calories and fat grams, measuring your food, etc. This is completely unnecessary if you will approach diet God's Weigh. God doesn't want you to waste your time in this way.

God's Weigh doesn't require anyone to push themselves to exhaustion to lose weight through lengthy and intense workouts, as glamorous an approach as this has become. If the Biggest Loser method was the right path, a contestant should be able to walk off the ranch, eat healthy, never embark on another focused exercise program, and still maintain their weight loss. Most fitness programs out these days support this 'beat the fat off your body' type of approach.

I do applaud The Biggest Loser for its efforts to encourage others to be physically active and to eat a healthy diet. I do believe that their intentions are good. But as far as the contestants go, the long-term value and sustainability of their weight loss and health is often sacrificed for entertainment value. Losing only a few pounds a week just isn't as exciting as 'double-digit' weight loss. And losing only a few pounds per week requires patience, an aspect of the fruit of the Spirit that is only available to Spirit-filled Believers.

I actually enjoy watching the show for its entertainment value, and I do love to see people lose weight. But I understand that The Biggest Loser process, at least as applied to its contestants, is no more a healthy path to weight loss than The Bachelor is to finding a marriage partner. It's predominately man's attempt to fix the problem through man's wisdom.

Despite what the wisdom of man regarding weight loss might say, an exercise program is completely unnecessary for weight loss. I reached my ideal body weight without any formal exercise whatsoever. Being physically active is certainly an important part of a healthy life long-term, but concentrated exercise is not a vital component for reaching your ideal body weight or healthy living.

Choosing the orange over the donut is the route to reaching your ideal body weight. Don't try to out-exercise an unhealthy diet. Don't try to work so hard that your inability to control your diet doesn't keep you from reaching your ideal body weight. This is not a good plan for long-term success. This is not God's Weigh to reach and maintain your ideal body weight.

I realize that embarking on an exercise program has seemingly become a moral matter these days. Working out is even seen as almost heroic. But the more I consider the fitness movement today, most especially as it pertains to intense exercise programs, the more clear does it show itself as a silly, foolish, big waste of time. I sense that the wildlife are looking at we humans and wondering if we have gone stark-raving mad.

I have heard it said that the only animal on the planet that moves more quickly when it is confused is the human. I think that is what we are seeing in today's fitness movement. There seems to be a new exercise regimen or piece of exercise equipment that comes out almost every day that promises to give you the perfect body. And then we have all the latest studies to help you determine the right fitness program for you.

There is no end to the clatter of everyone arguing that they have the solution to everyone's body weight problems. All the while, we just get fatter and fatter and fatter, much like their pocketbooks. Only a few have ever thought to stop the madness of it all, slow things down, and check in with God, the Creator of our bodies, to determine what He might suggest.

God is more concerned about your obedience to His Word than your willingness to sacrifice. Your willingness to sacrifice yourself to man-made exercise programs, exercise equipment, and diet plans will not get you to your ideal body weight in a sustainable way. But in God's Word will you will find God's Weigh, and it doesn't include intense, fat-burning cardio and strenuous, mass-building resistance training.

"… to obey is better than sacrifice…" (I Samuel 15:22, KJV)

The human tendency is to be willing to 'do more' when we set a goal of some sort. Trying to lose weight through an exercise program is a perfect example. Ultimately, most people approach a weight loss objective more from an 'exercise the fat off' angle, even though they might try to throw in a dietary improvement or two along the way.

The reason for this human tendency is that we want to live at our ideal body weights, but we don't want to give up our sodas, fried foods, and cookies. We are willing to 'do more' (exercise), but not really willing to 'require less' of anything (junk non-foods and/or excessive foods). We are willing to 'rely on our own efforts and plan,' but not really willing to 'rely on God's leading and wisdom.'

In my experience, and by what I read in Scripture about God, He appears to be a god who is more interested in having us learn to 'require less' (contentment, self-control, live a quiet and peaceable life, etc.) than to 'do more.' He appears to be a god more interested in having us learn to 'rely on His leading and wisdom' than to 'rely on our own efforts and plan.'

Man's way to overcome a problem or addiction is to cover it up, even if that means extra work. In this case, most had rather be told that God said we should run on the treadmill every day than to be told that God doesn't want us to eat refined sugars. We had rather do more work than to be required to depend upon God more, live with less, or have some pleasure taken from us.

God is not a god of 'doing more.' God is a god of 'requiring less,' of being 'controlled by less.' Consider this example. Let's say a man is earning $40K per year, but spending $45K per year. This is a financial problem, but more importantly, this is an indication of some underlying spiritual issue. What is man's way of trying to resolve the financial problem? He will often try to figure out a way to increase his earnings to the $45K he wants to spend. Think of 'earning more money' as analogous to exercise.

What will happen if this fellow figures out a way to increase his earnings to $45K? You guessed it. We will find him spending $50K. Why is that? This is because the underlying spiritual issue of the financial problem has not been addressed.

God's way, as well as the way that would be recommended by a wise financial advisor, would be for this man to learn to control his spending and live within his means first. And once he has mastered those various financial principles, then he can begin to consider ways to increase his earnings should he so desire. Think of 'spending money' as analogous to diet. God's way is for this guy to address his lack of control over his spending, not to determine how he can earn more money. And it is God's Weigh that you learn to walk in obedience to His dietary plan, not figure out a way to out-exercise a bad diet.

Man's approach doesn't address the underlying spiritual issues that have led to the weight gain. Man's approach is about getting the desired result that does not require spiritual growth. Man's way is not God's Weigh.

You will be much better off seeking to be physically active (as opposed to embarking on some exercise program); working in the yard, playing with your kids, walking your dog, hiking in the woods, helping a friend move, washing the car, playing golf, etc. My daughters were recently assigned a running regimen by their volleyball coach. I have joined them on some of those runs as a recreational outing. I look forward to doing the same with my grandkids someday. Living a happy and energetic life, a life that includes the purpose and plan that God will lead you towards, will provide you with more physical activity than you will ever need.

I recently saw a lady on television demonstrating some type of exercise program that revolved around performing certain common movements. I only caught a couple of them. One was 'clean the table' and the other was 'move and pull the piano'. You may have had this revelation yourself from other exercise programs that you have seen as well. It just tends to beg the question, 'Why not just go do those same movements while cleaning your house, rearranging your furniture, doing yard work, planting a garden, and so forth?' We pay someone else to do those things, and then we pay for a gym membership and/or exercise plan because there is not enough physical activity in our lives. That doesn't sound like God's economy to me.

There is just something instinctively questionable about a concentrated exercise program. There may be instances in which God could lead someone to embark on such training in order to complete some type of God-ordained mission, but for most of us, it is just a formula for self-focus and yet another addiction to add to our list. As I noted above, my daughters are required to complete several runs each week between volleyball practices as part of their conditioning for the sport. But this type of conditioning is obviously not required for the average adult.

If you are living a life that does not provide avenues to physical activity then I would contend that you are not living a good life to begin with. Stuffing in an exercise program at 5:00AM every morning or being away from your family with your 6:00PM, after-work sessions every evening is not the answer. Concentrated exercise programs are a waste of productive life. Live a meaningful, productive life and the exercise (physical activity) will be there.

You might think I am just someone who has never exercised (worked out) and doesn't know what I am talking about; some arm-chair quarterback on this subject. That is not the case. I was addicted to weightlifting for over 30 years. I have squatted 425 pounds for 5 reps. I have deadlifted 500 pounds. I have bench pressed 225 pounds for 11 reps. I have also run 5K, 10K, 15K, 20K, 25K, and marathon races. I have run 3 miles a day for 100 consecutive days.

I couldn't begin to calculate the thousands of hours I have spent (and wasted) in the form of formal exercise, along with all the planning, travel, and outfit-changing time. I take that back. Actually, I have estimated that total time for you. It comes out to over 10,500 total hours. To put this figure in more understandable terms, 10,500 hours equates to about 5 year's worth of full-time work (five 8-hour workdays per week) devoted to exercise program, focused time. It pains me to think of all that God could have accomplished in my life if I had given that time to Him.

I could hear the Holy Spirit's voice trying to speak to me at times during a workout. As I sat on the end of a bench, catching my breath between sets, I might look about the gym. I would watch others doing what I was doing. On numerous occasions the message that came to my mind was 'This is a foolish, self-focused, waste of time. What am I doing here?'

With the exception of a few brief periods of obedience along the way, I refused to heed this message. I think there were a couple of reasons why. One, exercise was, and had always been, an essential escape from the stress of life for me; howbeit the stress was because I was running from God. And two, I think that a part of me didn't want to acknowledge that I might have wasted decades of my life. In a sense, by keeping on with exercise, I continued to justify and validate its presence in my life for all those years.

Those 30 years of addictive exercise and self-focus kept me from God's best for my life. I know what I am talking about. Don't make the same mistake in your life.

Not only is an exercise program not necessary for you to reach your ideal body weight, but it could be the greatest diversion mankind ever created to keep you from seeking out and experiencing God's will for your life. I used exercise to escape from the pain I felt living a purposeless, meaningless life that had nothing to do with the way God created me and intended me to live. I used exercise to escape the voice of God, from His leading in my life. And I used exercise for my own vain, fleshly purposes.

And what did I get for all my formal exercise? I got 30 years wasted in an education and career that I cared nothing about. I got 30 years of not living in sync with God's will for my life. I got 30 years of unproductive, wasteful, painful time. I got a couple of bulging discs in my back and a couple of degenerative discs in my neck. I got tendinitis in my shoulders and elbows. Instead of others accepting me more, I found that it created a look and image that kept me separated from others; distinct in a cheesy, intimidating way. I missed out on so much 'living' as I did everything I could to escape from the pain of living a life apart from God's leading. Formal exercise has the potential of taking you out of one ditch (overweight) and putting you in a ditch that might even be worse. God doesn't mix blessing and cursing in this way.

"The blessing of the Lord, it maketh rich, and he addeth no sorrow with it." *(Proverbs 10:22, KJV)*

In my experience, I have actually found that direct, intense exercise seemed to work against my weight loss hopes. It may very well be because the high intensity that everyone promotes as required for progress and improvement (feel the burn, go for it, grit your teeth, no pain – no gain, and all that) creates such an incredible nutrient demand on the body through this self-applied stress that unless someone eats perfectly there will be more calories consumed than burned. For me, it seemed like for every 300 calories I might burn up through exercise I was probably consuming 500 calories of food trying to meet the nutritional deficiencies I created. That is why bodybuilders (which in affect I was) tend to bulk up during their mass-building cycle.

God makes a specific effort to downplay the importance of direct physical exercise in the Bible. God, the Creator of your body, took the time to minimize the value of direct physical exercise in your life. That is a huge statement. And it will be God who you must look to for all things fitness, this being the key to reaching your ideal body weight. Doing things God's Weigh (Godliness) will ensure your body is taken care of in the process, without a focused exercise program that primarily works to feed your flesh.

"But refuse profane and old wives' fables, and exercise thyself rather unto godliness. For bodily exercise profiteth little, but godliness is profitable unto all things, having the promise of the life that now is, and of that which is to come. This is a faithful saying..." (I Timothy 4:7-9, KJV)

This passage tells you that the importance put on direct physical exercise is a foolish practice. This passage tells you that God's leading in your life will not only take care of your physical requirements, but that all other components of your life will be made healthy as well. And this passage tells you that you can trust God on this one, not man. So spend your time focused on God's wisdom and leading in your life and all else will fall into place, without any exercise program. I Timothy 4:7-9 makes that very clear. An hour of Bible study and prayer will ultimately lead you to a healthier life - spiritually, emotionally, and physically - than an hour spent working an exercise program.

Such a direct focus on your physical body will feed your fleshly nature and not work to bring about the fruit of the Spirit in your life. That kind of inward, self-focus, at best, just gets you out of one ditch and over into another. You need a solution for the total person, without all of the negative side-effects.

It will be man's ways and wisdom that entice you with one promised benefit (if that) and several unknown (or not revealed) negative side-affects. God's ways are beneficial in all ways. Proverbs 10:22 (above) is a good acid test to apply to any philosophy that comes along your way to distract you from God's best for your life.

If you are still considering some type of exercise program, I would just encourage you to seek God's approval for what you should do, where you should do it, and the frequency and intensity with which you should do it. As I tried to point out above, a concentrated exercise program has the potential of taking you out of one ditch and putting you over into another, if not leaving you in both ditches at the same time for that matter.

For me, and I think for most, setting foot in a gym or working out to the latest exercise video is the last thing I should do relative to the health of my walk with God, and ultimately, the health of my body. Anything beyond a recreational walk/run and some basic calisthenics every now and then is most certainly an opportunity for the enemy to gain a foothold in your life.

Obedience is better than sacrifice, and more effective.

Five Spiritual Keys to Reaching Your Ideal Body Weight

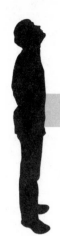
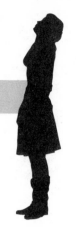

Chapter 5

Your Body is Not Your Own
& Dietary Disclaimer

There are five spiritual keys to reaching your ideal body weight. They are recognition of ownership, spiritual conditioning, leading of the Holy Spirit, purposeful living, and righteous motivation.

God's call for a dietary reformation in your life, and His desire for you to reach your ideal body weight, is not a call to you and God's people to become health nuts. This book is not about trying to convince you that you even need to be concerned about your health, body weight, and lifespan. This is my dietary disclaimer for this book.

As shocking as this may sound, it really doesn't matter whether or not you care about your physical health, your body weight, and how long you live. That 'care' will vary for you from day to day. There are plenty of people who will chose, and have chosen, to live unhealthy lives even though they know of the negative impact it will have on their health and lifespan. So a concern for your fitness level cannot and will not be what sustains you long-term. It will not be what enables you to both achieve and maintain your ideal body weight.

Although there is certainly nothing wrong with having a concern for your diet, body weight, and health, that isn't the motivation that will sustain you. God wants the best for you, whether you want the best for you or not. And we all know that what we want for ourselves, and what we are willing to do for what we want, changes with each passing day.

I would never want to waste my time, and yours, trying to convince you that you should be concerned about your health. I might be able to motivate you in some way for a time, but eventually, whether because of a bad day or just a general lack of concern, you will return to your unhealthy eating patterns. A concern for your health will not sustain you long-term.

There are people who have made the decision that they, regardless of the long-term consequences, would rather be left alone with their vices. Some people would, and have, made the choice to enjoy their unhealthy eating, alcohol, and tobacco over a more healthy and long life. Even for me, as someone who has an intellectual interest in fitness/physiology, without the daily acknowledgement that my body is not my own, there would be days I would choose unhealthy eating, alcohol, and tobacco over health.

What does matter to God, and therefore must matter to us as Christians, is that we walk in obedience to His commandments in every area of our lives, diet being one of those many areas. More specifically, you must recognize that your body is not your own, to treat in whatever manner you so decide on any given day. This is the mindset and motivation that will ensure your long-term success. This is the wisdom that the world of man's ways has completely missed, which of course it would. And unfortunately, the Church has operated by the same man-made wisdom.

It will be in recognizing that your body is not your own, to destroy with unhealthy living as you might desire, that you will reach your ideal body weight and maintain it. This point cannot be over-emphasized. Getting this settled in your mind will be one of the most fundamental keys to achieving your ideal body weight through Godly wisdom.

"What? Know ye not that your body is the temple of the Holy Ghost which is in you, which ye have of God, and ye are not your own? For ye are bought with a price: therefore glorify God in your body, and in your spirit, which are God's." (I Corinthians 6:19-20, KJV)

For me, a clear understanding and acknowledgement that my body was not my own was one of the top spiritual keys to success in walking in obedience to God's Word concerning diet and health, and reaching my ideal body weight.

I also found patience during the weight loss period as I accepted this truth. Even the world has determined that patience is essential to weight loss, and they happen to be right. Patience will come as you acknowledge that your body is God's. Confess that you messed up your body. But realize that now you have come to repentance and are moving forward with God's plan for your diet and health. There is a peace, a relief, and a patience that comes from just knowing you are now back on the right track, regardless of how long the trip might be. Walk forward in obedience and leave the results up to God.

There is another truth that should give you patience. You may not like this truth, but you need it. Although you will find a certain level of contentment with reaching and maintaining your ideal body weight, you must understand that reaching your ideal body weight is not the source of happiness. The only sustainable source of happiness will come from your relationship with God. So it is important that your joy come from walking in obedience to God's call on your life in this regard, not the end result. You can experience this joy from day one. You don't have to wait six months or more for the day when you finally reach your ideal body weight before you can have joy in the area of dietary holiness.

There were times I wanted to run to food because I had a sense of fear and anxiety about something, or I just really didn't care about my health and body weight on a particular day. What kept me from running to food (and junk non-foods) was to remind myself that my body was not my own. I actually found great relief in those 'giving over of my body to God' moments.

To recognize and accept that 'I did not have the right and freedom to harm my body' did so much for me in the way of removing the power of the temptation to eat in an unhealthy way. The 'restriction,' if you will, was actually 'freeing.' I think we find that to be true when we apply any directive from God. In one sense it is restrictive in that we should do this and we shouldn't do that per God's Word, but in reality, and ultimately, God's commandments prove to be quite freeing. This is a good point for those who would desire to believe that our freedoms in Christ have somehow freed us to harm our bodies in any way we so desire. The truth is that it is in giving in to God's commandments and directives for our lives that we find true freedom.

I see this truth played out in the process of parenting. Kids want what they want and are willing to fight for it, not knowing how harmful getting their way might be. We adults are not very different, usually just dressing up this tendency with the social graces we have developed over time.

What I have noticed was that when I battled with my children over something they wanted that was not good for them, and I did not give in, ultimately, a peace seemed to come over them. It wasn't that they wanted what they wanted any less, but what they gained from the process was a sense of peace in knowing that Dad was in control, that Dad was calling the shots, and that 'maybe' Dad wanted what was best for them. Deep down they needed to know that they were being held within the safety of their father's boundaries and control. In the restriction of not getting what they wanted they found freedom and peace.

Your body is not your own. Your heavenly Father is in control, is calling the shots, and wants the best for you. Within the restriction of accepting that your body is not your own, and obedience to God's dietary plan for your health and body weight, you will come to find emotional freedom and peace in living within those Godly boundaries. This is the kind of freedom that Jesus came to make available to us, not the freedom the Church claims it has to destroy our bodies with unhealthy living.

To be clear, what I have termed dietary disclaimer includes several defining characteristics. These include...

1) Understanding that developing a personal concern about diet, body weight, health, and lifespan is not God's primary objective for you, and is not the most important driver for you to achieve positive results in those areas of your life.

2) God wants you to experience your ideal body weight, good health, and a long lifespan, but God wants you to receive those blessings primarily through a focus on a desire and motivation to walk in obedience to His Word; the good fruit of that obedience (ideal body weight) being a natural by-product of that obedience.

3) God wants you to understand that your body is not your own, so it doesn't matter what concern you have for your body. Your body is God's business ultimately. Your concern for your health can vary from day to day, and that is okay. But your concern for your health is not what will sustain you.

4) There is nothing wrong with spending time meditating on the benefits of walking in obedience to God's Word concerning diet, it being a valuable secondary motivator for sure. But what you never want to waver on is your commitment to walking in obedience to God's Word. If you will let that be your primary driver you will not easily be knocked off course because today you care about your health, body weight, and lifespan, and tomorrow you don't.

I would not want the fact that this book addresses your dietary practices to leave you with a skewed Biblical perspective. The desire of God for this book, ministry, and message is not for you to develop a cultish focus in your life on physical health and your body. The underlying purpose of this book is to develop an overall focus on the importance of obedience to God's commandments, in this case, applied to the area of diet, body weight, and health.

As I will repeat several times throughout this book, I am not saying obedience to God's Word concerning diet and health is a requirement for salvation. That would be legalism to say so. But what I am saying is that dietary holiness is in fact a component of the holy and righteous life to which you are called as a Believer. This is your reasonable service. This is what God expects from His people. And God wants to bless you in the process.

"I beseech you therefore, brethren, by the mercies of God, that you present your bodies a living sacrifice, holy, acceptable to God, which is your reasonable service. And do not be conformed to this world, but be transformed by the renewing of your mind, that you may prove what is that good and acceptable and perfect will of God." (Romans 12:1-2, NKJV, BibleGateway.com)

Whether or not you are motivated by the benefits of obedience to God's commandments concerning diet is not the issue. What matters is that you acknowledge and obey His commandments. Period! This is your reasonable service.

Do not be conformed to the methods and motivations of this world, but rather, renew your mind with the wisdom and power of God's Word, proving in your life, for you and for the Church and for the world, what is the good, acceptable, perfect will of God. And you do this by offering your body as a living sacrifice to God. A tired, sick, and overweight body does not constitute an acceptable living sacrifice.

We need to seek and develop the desire to obey God's commands and to please Him. Obedience is what pleases God, not the fact that we may have figured out a way to become concerned about our diet, health, body weight, and lifespan. Focusing on staying in God's will, on track with His commands, is what will sustain you in your journey towards your ideal body weight.

You probably already know more about nutrition and its effect on the body than God ever thought necessary for you to know. There are plenty of books on the market that address the physical effects of diet; more are added to the list each year. Getting motivated by more study of nutritional insights and the latest diet and health studies will not sustain you. I tried that myself, with no lasting success.

Such information could be helpful if used properly. Understanding the destructive physical effects of refined sugars and overeating on the body, for example, could be used to help build your faith in the wisdom of God's dietary plan. Although knowing such information is not the truth you need, if you are wise, you can use it show the error of man's ways and to help point yourself and others to the truth. I will use some of those types of insights in this book.

Please allow the use of the term 'dietary disclaimer' and its defining characteristics to keep you steady on your journey towards your ideal body weight, and to help you maintain it; keeping you from getting knocked off track by those days and weeks where maintaining your ideal body weight matters less to you than your desire for soda, donuts, and fried chicken. Dietary disclaimer will be essential to ensuring that you do not lose 25, 50, 75, 100+ pounds during a season of high motivation regarding fitness, only to gain it back, and then some, when that motivation has waned.

Your body is not your own. The ownership goes to God. The responsibility for its care goes to you.

"Neither yield ye your members as instruments of unrighteousness unto sin: but yield yourselves unto God, as those that are alive from the dead, and your members as instruments of righteousness unto God." (Romans 6:13, KJV)

Chapter 6

Spiritual Conditioning is a Prerequisite to Physical Conditioning

There are five spiritual keys to reaching your ideal body weight. They are recognition of ownership, spiritual conditioning, leading of the Holy Spirit, purposeful living, and righteous motivation. The way we eat is one of the clearest reflections of our spiritual condition, yet is the most ignored.

What I refer to as spiritual conditioning is an absolute pre-requisite to true, lasting success in the area of physical conditioning that you seek; for success in anything for that matter. Spiritual conditioning goes beyond what you can derive from the intellectual knowledge of what you learn concerning diet, even that learned from the Bible.

It is not enough to just have intellectual knowledge regarding the truths of God's Word, you must exercise yourself unto a spiritually conditioned state whereby you are empowered to apply and follow through with that intellectual knowledge. Spiritual conditioning is the process of being filled with the Spirit.

Knowing more will not change your life. Without the spiritual strength to act on the things that you know, all the knowledge in the world (even Godly knowledge), will not have a lasting impact on your life. Spiritual conditioning is essential to reaching and maintaining your ideal body weight in a long-term, sustainable way.

There is a saturation in God's Word, prayer, worship, and progressive steps of obedience that creates a drunkenness, a filling, with the Spirit that makes doing the things of God a natural outflow. This is in contrast to drunkenness with wine that makes doing unsafe and unhealthy things a natural outflow.

"And be not drunk with wine, wherein is excess; but be filled with the Spirit." (Ephesians 5:18, KJV)

It is by direct Bible study, prayer, and worship, thereby enabling progressive obedience, that we achieve ever-increasing levels of spiritual conditioning in our lives; where we experience this 'filling with the Spirit' that makes obedience to God's dietary directives a natural outflow.

I have especially noticed the power of spiritual conditioning in my life in the area of forgiving and even blessing those who have wronged me. That is not a natural outflow of my flesh to say the least, which can be highly oriented towards bitterness and revenge; towards 'making things right' and 'settling the score.' On a side note, I have found that praying for the eternal salvation of those who have wronged me is one of the best ways to develop spiritual conditioning in my life. The difference between my desire to 'get them back' and a righteous concern for them is often a simple prayer to God, asking for their eternal salvation.

I do not believe that any book written about the Bible, even one loaded with Scripture references like this one, can provide the depth, width, and breadth of spiritual conditioning that direct Bible study and prayer offers.

You may never have heard the term spiritual conditioning, but you have probably heard of the fruit of the Spirit. Spiritual conditioning is what occurs as you actively seek to develop and apply the fruit of the Spirit to your life. The fruit of the Spirit is present in our lives when we are filled with the Spirit. And it is that constant filling with the Spirit through Bible study, prayer, worship, and progressive obedience that keeps us improving our spiritual conditioning.

"This I say then, Walk in the Spirit, and ye shall not fulfill the lust of the flesh. For the flesh lusteth against the Spirit, and the Spirit against the flesh: and these are contrary the one to the other; so that ye cannot do the things that ye would. But if ye be led of the Spirit, ye are not under the law. Now the works of the flesh are manifest, which are these; adultery, fornication, uncleanness, lasciviousness, Idolatry, witchcraft, hatred, variance, emulations, wrath, strife, seditions, heresies, Envying, murders, drunkenness, revellings, and such like: of the which I tell you before, as I have also told you in time past, that they which do such things shall not inherit the kingdom of God. But the fruit of the Spirit is love, joy, peace, longsuffering, gentleness, goodness, faith, Meekness, temperance: against such there is no law. And they that are Christ's have crucified the flesh with the affections and lusts. If we live in the Spirit, let us also walk in the Spirit." (Galatians 5:16-25, KJV)

It is fairly easy to see the many strengths that come with the fruit of the Spirit via spiritual conditioning. These strengths will be essential to enabling you to reach your ideal body weight through the faithful application of God's dietary plan. These strengths include long-suffering (patience is essential to the weight loss process as you very well and painfully know), goodness (dietary holiness), faith (that the application of God's Word will lead you to your ideal body weight), and temperance (self-control), as well as the support and presence of love, joy, and peace in your life.

It is worth noting that for some, self-control (part of the fruit of the Spirit / result of spiritual conditioning) is a more natural outflow of who they are, for a lack of a better way of saying it. For these people, the difference between walking in obedience to God's Word regarding diet and health, and not doing so, is simply learning what God's Word has to say about diet and health. For them, their primary issue is that they are just lacking the truth of God's Word concerning diet and health. They just didn't know any better; not that ignorance of God's Word is a valid excuse either.

My wife is largely this way. Self-control regarding diet is not a big struggle for her. All she needs to know is the truth of God's Word concerning diet and she is good to go.

While for others, like me, spiritual conditioning, this filling with the Spirit, is absolutely essential to success in the area of diet and health. The very fact that I am writing this book and you are reading it tells me that you and I have tendencies towards fleshly lusts concerning our diets. All the dietary wisdom in the world, even Biblical dietary wisdom, is not enough, in and of itself, to strengthen me to obedience.

I wish knowledge was enough alone, because I tend to be an intellectual; extensively studying and learning whatever subject matter has caught my attention or in which I know I need help. I am not lacking in Biblical wisdom in most cases, just the spiritual power to follow through with it. I probably know more about what I 'should be doing' than what I 'am doing' than anybody on the planet. I need that constant filling of the Spirit, that spiritual conditioning, in order to walk in obedience to God's Word concerning diet and health.

I think it best to play it safe and assume that you are the same as me in this regard. In any event, God requires that we all be filled with the Spirit. This is not a suggestion and there are no exceptions. And besides, although one person may have a tendency towards ease of self-control with their dietary practices, they may not have that same natural tendency towards self-control in other areas of their lives; say in the area of finances or gossip, for example.

I could spend the rest of this book telling you what to eat and what not to eat (and I will get to that later). This information would be the more technical do's and don'ts aspect of achieving success in the area of reaching your ideal body weight. But is that what you really need? Is that information the key to your breakthrough, to reaching your ideal body weight? You already know the answer... NO. You already know ten times more about healthy living now than you are successfully applying to your life as it is.

That being said, I must say that I do believe you will be impacted and amazed as you see that God's Word does in fact speak to the technical do's and don'ts of your diet and health. But even with those insights you will still need spiritual conditioning to follow through with doing what you know to be right and avoiding those things you know to be wrong; that battle of the Spirit (life) verses your flesh (death).

"It is the Spirit who gives life; the flesh profits nothing. The words that I speak to you are spirit, and they are life." (John 6:63, NKJV, BibleGateway.com)

"For to be carnally minded is death, but to be spiritually minded is life and peace." (Romans 8:6, NKJV, BibleGateway.com)

"For he who sows to his flesh will of the flesh reap corruption, but he who sows to the Spirit will of the Spirit reap everlasting life." (Galatians 6:8, NKJV, BibleGateway.com)

To 'sow' to something simply means to make decisions in favor of that something. Every time you make the decision to eat an orange rather than a donut, you have sown to your Spirit (life and strength) and not to your flesh (death and weakness). In doing this you have strengthened your spiritual power (spiritual conditioning) and weakened the power of your flesh over your future decisions.

"This I say then, Walk in the Spirit, and ye shall not fulfill the lust of the flesh. For the flesh lusteth against the Spirit, and the Spirit against the flesh: and these are contrary the one to the other; so that ye cannot do the things that ye would." (Galatians 5:16-17, KJV)

Relative to reaching your ideal body weight, you already know to drink water instead of soda. You already know to eat your fruits and vegetables instead of candies and desserts. You already know to eat grilled chicken instead of fried chicken. You already know to stop eating when you are full. You already know not to eat just because you are bored or sad.

You know that you are not overweight due to a lack of dietary technical knowledge. Stop living in denial of that reality as you read diet book after diet book looking for some magic pill of technical knowledge that will allow you to still live any way you want and achieve the results you desire. I have been guilty of that. Although there is no magic pill in the area of technical knowledge, there is a magic pill relative to the power to succeed. And it's called spiritual conditioning; achieved through daily Bible study, prayer, and worship, followed by progressive steps of obedience.

Please do not misunderstand me. I will provide you with some excellent Biblical wisdom/techniques for obtaining your ideal body weight. That is ahead, and you will be amazed as to what God has to say about the subject. But what I am saying is that you can have all the technical knowledge available (even Biblically sound technical knowledge), but it is of little value if you do not have the strength, or what I call spiritual conditioning, necessary to put that technical knowledge into practice.

The importance of spiritual conditioning comes from the fact that we wrestle not with flesh and blood, but against spiritual wickedness. Mental knowledge and human determination are no match against the forces of spiritual wickedness that seek to keep you from good health and your ideal body weight. You cannot fight those evil forces with your own power and might. You need the power and might of God to be victorious in such a battle.

"Finally, my brethren, be strong in the Lord, and in the power of his might. Put on the whole armour of God, that ye may be able to stand against the wiles of the devil. For we wrestle not against flesh and blood, but against principalities, against powers, against the rulers of the darkness of this world,

against spiritual wickedness in high places. Wherefore take unto you the whole armour of God, that ye may be able to stand in the evil day, and having done all, to stand. Stand therefore, having your loins girt about with truth, and having on the breastplate of righteousness; And your feet shod with the preparation of the gospel of peace; Above all, taking the shield of faith, wherewith ye shall be able to quench all the fiery darts of the wicked. And take the helmet of salvation, and the sword of the Spirit, which is the word of God: Praying always…" (Ephesians 6:11-18, KJV)

Notice the similar elements/strengths found in the 'armor' required for victory and the fruit of the Spirit… truth (God's dietary plan), righteousness (goodness / dietary holiness), patience (long-suffering), faith (faith), and God's Word (the source of God's dietary plan). This passage also points to the fact that this victory is only available to those who have accepted Jesus Christ as their Savior (salvation). It also points to the fact that prayer will be critical to winning this spiritual battle in your life.

Again spiritual conditioning is achieved only through Bible study, prayer, and worship, followed by progressive steps of obedience that have thereby been enabled. The progressive steps of obedience play an important part in that good actions tend towards more good actions, while bad actions tend towards more bad actions. But please be clear that Bible study, prayer, and worship are foundational even to those progressive steps of obedience. The number one exercise for weight loss is a daily regimen of Bible study, prayer, and worship.

There is a good analogy (or bad as the case may be) of this spiritual conditioning principle, which unfortunately is exactly the way most Christians approach their Christian walk. Let's consider the goal of running a successful marathon (not that God is calling anyone to do so).

You could spend countless hours studying the various technical aspects of successfully running a marathon, and I have. You may learn of the importance of maintaining a 180-step per minute cadence, the benefits of running the race in a negative split format, a recommended training plan that includes a portfolio of short fast runs and longer slow runs, etc. But if you walk up to the starting line on race day without having exercised your physical body and think you can grit your teeth through to a successful run with just that technical knowledge, you are crazy.

Why? Because you have not conditioned your body to follow through with the technical knowledge that you have obtained. No one would ever do that (relative to a foot-race), but we see the Christian community facing their life challenges in exactly the same way; gaining some technical knowledge on a subject (maybe even Biblical technical knowledge) and expecting to grit their teeth through to success without having exercised themselves spiritually (spiritual conditioning) through consistent Bible study, prayer, and worship.

Spiritual conditioning will spell the difference between success and failure in your journey to reach and maintain your ideal body weight.

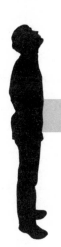
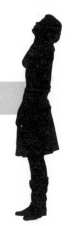

Chapter 7

The Holy Spirit Leading You to Your Ideal Body Weight

There are five spiritual keys to reaching your ideal body weight. They are recognition of ownership, spiritual conditioning, leading of the Holy Spirit, purposeful living, and righteous motivation.

If you have struggled with your weight you may find the subject matter in this chapter offensive. In this chapter we will address the value of shame in our lives. Although it is certainly not my intent to offend anyone, but to help, the truth itself can have that effect at times. And it will be the truth, even painful truth, that will work to set you free from bondage to unhealthy eating and help you reach your ideal body weight. Please consider this chapter the 'tough love' chapter.

As you read through this chapter I think you will come to realize that the offense you feel comes from your prideful flesh and/or a lack of Biblical insight into the value of shame in your life. Also, you will come to realize that the shame of being overweight is not an issue of self-respect and self-esteem, but simply the Holy Spirit trying to work in your life to bring you to a better place.

"For I know the thoughts that I think toward you, saith the Lord, thoughts of peace, and not of evil..." (Jeremiah 29:11, KJV)

And just to be clear before moving forward, I am not saying that there is no such thing as unfounded shame; that is, shame based on an incorrect belief / perspective. For example, a child of divorced parents might be ashamed of themselves because they believe their parents' divorce was their fault. This child's shame is founded on an incorrect belief / perspective. That is not what I am I talking about here. So when I use the word shame in this book I am referring to a righteous shame, a God-ordained shame if you will.

It is the Holy Spirit's job to help guide and direct you away from unhealthy practices (lack of dietary holiness), and their resulting bad fruit (overweight or underweight), that you may have unknowingly, or knowingly, embarked upon.

"If you love Me, keep My commandments. And I will pray the Father, and He will give you another Helper, that He may abide with you forever the Spirit of truth, whom the world cannot receive, because it neither sees Him nor knows Him; but you know Him, for He dwells with you and will be in you." (John 14:15-17, NKJV, BibleGateway.com)

The Holy Spirit is the Spirit of Truth working in you as a Believer. That is huge. Whether you are spending time in Bible study and prayer or not, and whether you are walking in obedience to God's Word or not, there is always the Holy Spirit poking His spotlight around inside of you to highlight any sin that may be present in your life.

There is no escape from the scrutiny of the Holy Spirit in your life, as hard as you might try to find one. Maybe that escape is food for you. Could it be that your addiction to food, or any addiction in the life of the Believer, is primarily an attempt to cover up the pain caused by your resistance to the leading of the Holy Spirit?

Is the Holy Spirit telling you to get out of a bad relationship, that he/she is no good for you? Is the Holy Spirit telling you that your choice of career paths was only about money, not about what God wants you to do with your life? Is the Holy Spirit telling you to forgive someone or ask for forgiveness, but you refuse? And then could you be running to food to quench the working and message of the Holy Spirit within you, because you have refused to listen and obey His leading?

"Quench not the Spirit." (I Thessalonians 5:19, KJV)

Are you quenching the Holy Spirit's workings within you with unhealthy dietary practices? Are you using food to drown out the voice of the Holy Spirit inside you? What message are you running from?

Don't quench the Spirit with addictive behaviors. Obedience and the resulting freedom you will find in giving in to the Holy Spirit's leading in your life is so much better than what unhealthy eating can offer. I think (I know) this is a foundational issue relative to addictive behaviors in the life of the Believer. And this is an issue that you will need to address in your life as you seek to reach your ideal body weight. Find out what the Holy Spirit is leading you to do and do it!!! Your ability to control your diet and reach your ideal body weight depends on it.

I hope you will agree that the diligent study of God's Word is part of His will for your life. We often struggle with our search for God's will in our lives, but neglect those aspects of His will that are plainly stated in Scripture. In studying God's Word we can gain some helpful insights into His will and purpose for shame in our lives.

"Study to show thyself approved unto God, a workman that needeth not to be ashamed, rightly dividing the word of truth." (II Timothy 2:15, KJV)

Notice the word 'ashamed' in this verse. If you are 25, 50, 75, or 100+ pounds overweight, I think it would be safe to say that you may feel ashamed of it. You instinctively know that there is something wrong in your life. I am not trying to throw salt in your wound by highlighting this point. I want to help you, and this is an important place for us to touch upon as you travel down the pathway to your ideal body weight.

For those of you who have not been at your ideal body weight in decades, if ever in your life, reaching your ideal body weight will feel like 'coming home.' You will know that living your life at your ideal body weight is an important part of who you were always meant to be. You will feel like you are the correct representation of who God intended for you to be. It will feel so right. I want to give you this hope as you work through the challenging days of spiritual battle ahead. It will all be worth it to get back to a 'home' you may have never been to before.

Shame is not to be ignored, denied, or set aside. Shame is to be carefully considered to determine weaknesses in your life that need to be corrected. Shame is the natural consequence of walking in disobedience to God's Word, for not rightly dividing and applying the 'word of truth' in your life. And do not despise the chastening of the Lord and the leading of the Holy Spirit in your life, but begin to walk in obedience to His commands.

"My son, despise not the chastening of the Lord, neither be weary of his correction; for whom the Lord loveth he correcteth, even as a father the son in whom he delighteth." (Proverbs 3:11-12, KJV)

And by the way, shame, through the conviction of the Holy Spirit, can exist whether or not those consequences show up on the outside for others to see. Sinful dietary practices, unlike a lot of other sinful behaviors, produce consequences (excess weight) that cannot be hidden. I think that is why unhealthy eating is the Church's 'drug of choice,' our 'secret sin' as the Bible often refers to this type of struggle in our lives. We cannot hide the consequences of an unhealthy diet because of the excess weight that is often produced.

We know that unforgiveness is wrong, but we think we can hide it. We know that not loving our spouse is wrong, but we think we can hide it. We know that materialism is wrong, but we think we can hide it. We know that sexual lust is wrong, but we think we can hide it. But you know you cannot hide the consequences (excess weight) of walking in disobedience to God's Word concerning diet and health. In a sense, it puts disobedience to God's dietary directives in its own special category.

This is why the Church will preach about forgiveness, love, materialism, and even sexual lust, and we won't squirm in the pews too much. But the Church has shown that it doesn't want to touch dietary holiness. As a matter of fact, the Church has successfully worked to misinterpret Scripture, improperly define and misapply Bible principles, and convince itself that there is no such thing as dietary holiness, and to even speak of it is legalism. This is a characteristic of the dietary deception that Satan has so successfully achieved in our midst through the cooperation of our fleshly desires.

The Church doesn't seem to even know how to correctly define legalism, much less correctly apply it. Legalism, by example, is not communicating that God has a standard for holy living, to include with respect to our dietary practices. Legalism is arguing that holy living is a requirement for salvation. No one is arguing that dietary holiness is a requirement for salvation. We are saved by grace, and grace alone.

"For by grace are ye saved through faith; and that not of yourselves: it is a gift of God." (Ephesians 2:8, KJV)

The world tries to tell you that shame is something to be overcome with positive thinking, that your shame is a lack of self-respect and self-esteem. The world tells you that you need to develop a mindset that convinces you to accept your body just the way it is, thereby overcoming that lack of self-respect and self-esteem.

This 'wisdom' is not unlike reducing the level of difficulty of academic testing in the government school system in an effort to keep from 'damaging the self-esteem' of the children. The real issue is that the children who might fail the test have not 'studied to show themselves approved' by way of a passing grade. And consequently, they will experience shame. This is a good thing. This is a God thing. We need to allow shame to do its work in our lives and in the lives of our children.

Those kids who did not study and subsequently failed the test, they are in need of reproof, correction, and instruction. If you are overweight then you are also in need of reproof, correction, and instruction, that you might be perfect and thoroughly furnished unto all good works; that you might live your life at your ideal body weight.

"All scripture is given by inspiration of God, and is profitable for doctrine, for reproof, for correction, for instruction in righteousness: That the man of God may be perfect, thoroughly furnished unto all good works." (II Timothy 3:16-17, KJV)

"Poverty and shame shall be to him that refuseth instruction; but he that regardeth reproof shall be honored." (Proverbs 13:18, KJV)

God tells us that shame is a red-flag that something is wrong in our lives. Don't turn off God's alarm with worldly wisdom. That is Satan's strategy to keep you from the life God wants for you; to keep you from your ideal body weight.

Shame is the alarm that the Holy Spirit will sound in your heart when you have gone astray. Trying to gain a positive mindset to overcome the shame you feel is like turning off the fire alarm and thinking you have resolved the emergency, even though your building is still on fire. Turning off the fire alarm doesn't help a thing. As a matter of fact, turning off the fire alarm will only work to ensure greater potential damage to the building, to you, and to others.

If you try to turn off the alarm of shame, then your unhealthy diet will be allowed to continue to destroy and burn away at the quality of your life, the value of your life to God's work and God's plan for you, and your pursuit of your ideal body weight. Don't waste your life in this way.

Shame will highlight bad actions and bad fruit in your life. The Holy Spirit will use shame to direct you back to God and the 'straight and narrow'; calling you to repentance for the sinful ways that have brought you to an unhealthy body weight.

"For a good tree does not bear bad fruit, nor does a bad tree bear good fruit. For every tree is known by its own fruit..." (Luke 6:43-44, NKJV, BibleGateway.com)

God's people are called to live a life above reproach and free from all appearances of evil. We know that a lack of dietary holiness in our lives leads to poor health and excess weight. This is anything but living a life above reproach. And to be overweight most certainly carries with it the appearance of evil.

"Abstain from all appearance of evil." (I Thessalonians 5:22, KJV)

There is something I have observed over the years regarding someone's appearance. A person's appearance can affect how they are treated. That is probably not a grand revelation for most. We all know that a clean, well-dressed person will tend to garner more respect and favor than someone who is unkept and poorly dressed. But there are other ways in which a person's appearance can affect how they are treated.

I will use men in this example because I think it may apply more often to men than women. All things being the same, the taller of two men will garner more immediate respect and favor than the shorter man. We know that King Saul was much taller than his fellow man; a trait that was attributable to much of the favor he enjoyed.

This is a cold hard fact of life. And at only 5'8" tall myself, I wish it weren't true. I have said at times 'For every inch shorter in height, you have to be 10% more of a man to get the same results in life.' I realize this statement is not how the Christian person should view life. God's plans for each of our lives will most certainly supersede the influence of a person's height. But nevertheless, the reality of this difference in perception regarding height plays out every day.

I can remember a tall man, about 6'6" tall, telling me that he has enjoyed many professional opportunities simply because of his height. All things being the same, the 5'6" guy had better have a whole lot more on the ball than the 6'2" guy to get the job, get the break, or get the whatever. That is not to say that many shorter men have not done things far greater than other much taller men, but as far as a first impression goes, this seems to be the case. This is truly unfair, most especially because a person cannot control their height. But is making a judgment based on appearance always unfair, even wrong, especially when it is relative to something that can be changed or controlled?

If you are overweight, you may have felt unfairly treated. Someone else got the job, got the girl/guy, got the friends, got the respect, and got the breaks because you were overweight. If this is how you were made to feel, you probably also felt bitter and resentful about it. You may have perceived this as prejudice and unfair treatment. Although I would never commend rude and unfair treatment of anyone, is this really unfair treatment or is it the natural consequence of sin? Let me explain.

I once had an employee who smoked regularly. I will call him by the name of John. John would routinely take smoke breaks. He also traveled from company site to company site as part of his maintenance duties, which enabled him to smoke as he drove along as well. I tried to discourage John from smoking.

I would tell John 'Let's say we had three maintenance employees; one that smoked and two that didn't. If the company determined that we needed to downsize to only two maintenance employees, which employee do you think would be targeted for elimination? Even if the productivity of all three employees was the same, the one targeted would be the smoker.'

Is that a show of prejudice and unfairness, or is it a demonstration of discernment by management? You see, whether John liked it or not, and whether his productivity was lower than the others or not, smoking is perceived as a weakness, and rightfully so.

A quick aside – The Church has actually come down on those who smoke, howbeit an unwritten standard for acceptabe conduct. That is a good thing. But the Church has continued to maintain its one drug of choice, unhealthy eating. By comparison, I would contend that one 12-ounce soda is as damaging to your health as 2 to 3 cigarettes. What would be more damaging to your body, a pack of cigarettes each day or 7 to 10 sodas each day? It is something for the Church, with soda and donut in hand, to think about the next time it looks down its nose at a smoker.

The image that a smoker tends to project to their employer and others is that they are not wise, lack self-control, may tend too much to their fleshly desires and not enough to their work, do not project a positive company image, will waste more time with breaks than the non-smoker, and will ultimately be less productive. Is that true in every case? No. But is that wise discernment on the part of the employer? I would contend, yes.

Change the person involved in this scenario from someone who smokes to someone who is overweight. Does the image of an overweight person project to their employer and others that they are not wise, lack self-control, may tend too much to their fleshly desires and not enough to their work, do not project a positive company image, will waste more time with breaks than someone who is not overweight, and will ultimately be less productive? Yes. Is that true in every case? No. But is that wise discernment on the part of the employer? I would again contend, yes.

I would further contend that this is Godly wisdom on the part of the employer. God's Word supports the need for concern on behalf of the employer.

"Their destiny is destruction, their god is their stomach, and their glory is in their shame. Their mind is on earthly things." (Philippians 3:19, NIV)

"Poverty and shame shall be to him that refuseth instruction; but he that regardeth reproof shall be honored." (Proverbs 13:18, KJV)

By the way, there is a tendency for some fleshly issues to begat other fleshly issues in the case of some people. The more they give in to one fleshly issue the more they tend to give into another. In John's case, his combo was smoking and an extremely unhealthy diet, along with alcohol in past years.

I would confide in my boss in that I would be surprised if John made it past the age of 55. As it turned out, he didn't quite make it to 50, dying six months before due to a combination of unhealthy eating, tobacco, and previous years of alcohol abuse. John looked like he was nine-months pregnant when he died (visceral fat, which I will discuss later). Don't let this be your future and reputation. Don't let this be the legacy you leave for your children to follow. Don't let this be your witness to the world of what the wisdom and power of God's Word can do.

Don't let fleshly pride be the downfall to you reaching your ideal body weight. You must take responsibility for the consequences of the actions in your life that have brought you to the point of being overweight and all the pain and baggage that has come with it.

"Pride goes before destruction, and a haughty spirit before a fall." (Proverbs 16:18, NKJV, BibleGateway.com)

"… God resisteth the proud…" (James 4:6, KJV)

It may very well be that being overweight for you is the result of anything but a lack of self-respect and self-esteem. Could it be more through a spirit of pride in your life that you have found yourself at this place? I think this might give some a lot to prayerfully consider.

The problem is not in how the world perceives and reacts to those who are overweight. Although the specific ways in which they react, whether kind or unkind may vary, the harsh reality is that an inability to control your diet and body weight is a weakness that cannot be hidden; a weakness the world will not show respect and favor towards.

Would an adulterer be treated with the same type of prejudice if found out? Yes. Would someone who was unkind to his wife and children be treated with the same type of prejudice if found out? Yes. Would someone who was known to cheat on their taxes be treated with the same type of prejudice if found out? Yes. Unfortunately, or fortunately as the case may be, being overweight has the potential of receiving the greatest outward pressure for improvement due to the negative reactions from those around us. But because so many of us are still overweight, we have evidently determined some way to live in denial of this reality and pressure. Maybe that is why we work so hard to protest how others treat us. We don't want to see that the problem is us.

You must understand the shame you feel regarding your excess weight is the pressure that is working on the inside of you. The perception and discernment of others regarding your condition is pressure working from the outside. Both are the consequences of the same thing; failure to walk in obedience to God's dietary directives and to achieve your ideal body weight.

Shame is a result of the Holy Spirit working within you to bring you to an ever-increasing level of holy living; to shine the light on an area of sin in your life. You are not struggling with an issue of self-esteem, but rather a resistance to the leading of the Holy Spirit.

I know this has been a difficult discussion. But if you will allow it, the pain and shame you are feeling can be a very important part of your journey to your ideal body weight. This is an example of where 'no pain – no gain' is Biblically supported.

Please close out this chapter by carefully and prayerfully meditating over the following Scriptures; considering the discussion above, how these verses apply to your disobedience to God's dietary directives, why you are overweight, and how shame is an indication that something needs to change.

If you will follow God's dietary directives you will find that you will no longer have to live in shame regarding your excess bodyweight. You will be able to reach and maintain your ideal body weight. You will be a 'workman that needeth not to be ashamed' if you will obey His commands.

"O that my ways were directed to keep thy statutes! Then shall I not be ashamed, when I have respect unto all thy commandments." (Psalm 119:5-6, KJV)

I want to end this chapter with a number of verses that address shame. These are extremely hard-hitting; nothing held back. But please understand that I did not write them. The God that loves you wrote them. And He believes these messages to be the best way to help you. This is God's 'tough love.'

"The wise shall inherit glory, but shame shall be the promotion of fools." (Proverbs 3:35, KJV)

"The righteous hate what is false, but the wicked bring shame and disgrace." (Proverbs 13:5, KJV)

"We lie down in our shame, and our confusion covereth us; for we have sinned against the Lord our God, we and our fathers, from our youth even unto this day, and have not obeyed the voice of the Lord our God." (Jeremiah 3:25, KJV)

"O Lord, we and our kings, our princes and our fathers are covered with shame because we have sinned against you." (Daniel 9:8, KJV)

"... the one who trusts in Him will never be put to shame." (Romans 9:33, KJV)

"Come back to your senses as you ought, and stop sinning; for there are some who are ignorant of God – I say this to your shame." (I Corinthians 15:34, KJV)

"Rather, we have renounced secret and shameful ways; we do not use deception, nor do we distort the word of God. On the contrary, by setting forth the truth plainly we commend ourselves to every man's conscience in the sight of God." (II Corinthians 4:2, KJV)

"To my shame I admit that we were too weak for that!" (II Corinthians 11:21, KJV)

"Many will follow their shameful ways and will bring the way of truth into disrepute." (II Peter 2:2, KJV)

"Proving what is acceptable unto the Lord. And have no fellowship with the unfruitful works of darkness, but rather reprove them. For it is a shame even to speak of those things which are done of them in secret. But all things that are reproved are made manifest by the light: for whatsoever doth make manifest is light. Wherefore he saith, Awake thou that sleepest, and arise from the dead, and Christ shall give thee light. See then that ye walk circumspectly, not as fools, but as wise, Redeeming the time, because the days are evil. Wherefore be ye not unwise, but understanding what the will of the Lord is." (Ephesians 5:10-17, KJV)

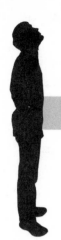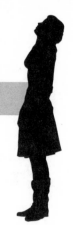

Chapter 8

The Pursuit of Purpose Creates a Better Life Than The Pursuit of Pleasure

There are five spiritual keys to reaching your ideal body weight. They are recognition of ownership, spiritual conditioning, leading of the Holy Spirit, purposeful living, and righteous motivation.

Living life without a Godly purpose and focus is an incredible source of stress and pain for the Believer. I know what it means to dread day after day after day of purposeless living; dragging myself off to a meaningless job day in day out, week in week out, month in month out, year in year out.

How did I try to cope with the pain of such a life? The same way many Believers try to endure such a meaningless life. If your life isn't about purpose it will be about the pursuit of pleasure in the form of addictive behaviors. It is just that simple. We will either seek God and His plan for our lives or we will live our lives in the pursuit of pleasure, or more aptly put, escape.

Depending upon the individual, this addictive, pleasure-seeking mindset can seek relief from the pain of purposeless living from many sources. Some of those include food and junk non-foods, alcohol, tobacco, gambling, sexual lust, materialism/money, the obsessive need for approval from others, fame, power, control, gossip, and computer gaming, to name some of the more common addictive tendencies.

King Solomon can tell you what a life lived out in the pursuit of pleasure will bring.

"I said in mine heart, Go to now, I will prove thee with mirth… laughter… wine… pleasure… great works… gardens… pools… servants… great possessions… silver and gold… I was great…" (Ecclesiastes 2:1-9, KJV)

This list looks like the same list of things many people in modern America are pursuing. What did King Solomon get for his pursuit of pleasure?

"… I hated life…" (Ecclesiastes 2:17, KJV)

The pain of a life spent in the pursuit of pleasure will leave you miserable. Does this describe your experience with unhealthy eating? Has your addiction to unhealthy eating, your pursuit of pleasure, brought you to the point where life is simply miserable? If so, then the solution is changing your life focus from a pursuit of pleasure to a pursuit of purpose.

Where does the pain of purposeless living come from? It comes from the same place as the shame of being overweight that we discussed earlier, the Holy Spirit. Although I am sure non-believers would prefer a purposeful life, I don't believe it is as critical to their emotional stability as it is for the Believer. I wouldn't expect a non-believer to be overly happy, but I would expect that they can more easily drown themselves in meaningless activity and worldly motivations with less of a tendency for pause and concern.

As Believers we have the Holy Spirit indwelling us. And the Holy Spirit can't stand a wasted and unfruitful life. The Holy Spirit is all about having us live a purposeful life walked out in obedience to God and service to others. If we are not pursuing a purposeful life we will be miserable. And either we will turn to God to resolve the source of our misery or we will attempt to escape this pain through pleasure.

The Holy Spirit of God is constantly harassing us over our purposeless living. This means that we will listen to God's voice through the leading of the Holy Spirit, and begin walking in obedience to His directives, or we will pick one or more of the addictive behaviors listed above to drown Him out; to quench the work of the Holy Spirit in our lives.

"Quench not the Spirit." (I Thessalonians 5:19, KJV)

Why would anybody ever want to quench the voice of God in their lives? I think in large part it is an issue of fear. At its core, we are afraid that what God has to offer will not be as pleasing as what we have come up with for a life. And the strange thing is that we can maintain this fear and belief even when we are miserable. Such is the power of Satan to deceive and destroy everything that is good; everything that God wants for His people.

I have been an expert at quenching the Spirit over the course of my life, ever since I became a Christian at the age of eleven. I quenched the Spirit through a variety of addictive behaviors. One of the addictive behaviors whereby I quenched the Holy Spirit's work in my life was through weightlifting. I was obsessed with weightlifting and bodybuilding. During high-school I finally got the attention that I always wanted. But after high-school, through college and throughout adulthood, it became my escape.

I can still hear my mom's voice saying 'I don't know why you think you have to lift those old weights.' It is funny, saddening really, when we can recall a comment made by a coach, a teacher, or a parent like that. The sad part is that we never take it enough to heart at the time. It took be about 20 years to finally 'get it,' but it was another 10 years (30 years total) before I finally set the weights down, before I submitted to God's leading in that regard.

I didn't participate in basketball, baseball, and track my Junior and Senior years in high-school because I was so addicted to weightlifting and bodybuilding that I feared those activities would take away from my progress. That was such a tragedy in my life. I loved sports and I was a very good athlete.

I did play football, but that was more because the unspoken message in my small town was 'you aren't one of the guys and you are one of the odd people if you don't play football.' So as a young kid and teenager, I had no choice but to respond to that kind of pressure. But I would still lift weights during my free period before afternoon practice.

I would literally break into the school gym on weekends so I could lift weights. I didn't actually break anything. I could usually find an unlocked window to crawl in. I am still a pretty determined person, but these days I am directing my determination towards Godly and purposeful living. There is such a massive difference between an enslavement to which you will answer at all costs, and the freedom of living a life determined to walk in obedience to the Holy Spirit's leading in your life.

"…let us lay aside every weight, and the sin which doth so easily beset us, and let us run with the patience the race that is set before us…" (Hebrews 12:1, KJV)

It is interesting that for me, 'laying aside every weight' in order to move forward with God's best for my life involved a literal 'laying aside of the weights.'

Similarly, I remember one day in high-school chemistry class, my teacher took a break from the normal routine to discuss college with us Seniors. She asked what each of was planning on studying in college. My answer was 'Engineering, because engineers make a lot of money.' She paused, looked at me carefully the way all good teachers seem to be able, and said 'All the money in the world won't matter if you aren't happy with what you are doing.' Like my mother's voice, I could hear those words echoing in the back of my mind for 30 years before they finally helped to result in positive fruit in my life.

Maybe someone has spoken something special into your life; a parent, a teacher, a coach, or your pastor. And maybe the Holy Spirit is echoing their words off the walls of your mind, but they have not come to any good fruit as of yet in your life. Stop now, listen closely, and carefully consider what messages God is trying to send you through the people and leaders He has placed in your life. And please do it before you waste 30 years of your life!

I hated my field of study in college. I was the furthest thing from an engineer anyone could possibly be. I can remember days when I would look out the classroom window at other students walking about campus, feeling like I was imprisoned, with no hope of escape.

But I still made the grades, being so determined to succeed and to impress as I was. I was addicted to making A's and addicted to receiving praise from my coaches and teachers. I used that addiction to drown out the leading of the Holy Spirit in my life throughout college. I ended up with a GPA of 3.8, Summa Cum Laude, in a field of study that I hated. I couldn't stop. I thought that would be quitting, and I could never be known as a quitter. Yes, I was a big ball of issues.

So how did I survive college, failing to ever submit to the direction of the Holy Spirit along the way? Of course, I held tight to my addictive weightlifting and bodybuilding. But then I also added alcohol on the weekends. I firmly believed, and in a sense it was true, that I had to have the escape of alcohol to survive my miserable college experience.

After college, I added unhealthy eating (that was actually present all along to varying degrees). I hated my work. I needed more frequent escapes than weightlifting and alcohol could offer me, so I added gluttonous and unhealthy eating to the list. For me to even act like I was interested in the job during the interview process was worthy of an Academy Award, and I had to fake interest each and every day after. I know what it means to get to the point where I could say that food was my only friend, at least the only friend the Church would allow.

I eventually added tobacco to my ever-growing list of vices. An addictive spirit cannot be satisfied. It is a bottomless pit; a fire that cannot be quenched. It just grows and grows and grows, along with a person's body weight eventually.

I looked like the picture of perfect health on the outside from the weightlifting and bodybuilding training, while I was destroying my body on the inside with late-night study, hard weekend living, and an unhealthy diet. It wasn't until I hit about thirty that the bad fruit of my bad ways began to show up on my waistline. You can only out-run a bad diet for just so long.

I think the aging process is an example of God's long-suffering and patience, and an example of the sanctification process He intends for all Believers. With each passing year we gradually become less able to get away with our sinful ways, at least not without consequences that become unacceptable and intolerable to us. In that process God patiently and effectively works to get our attention, although some of us are more stubborn than others. That's a book for another day.

I know everyone talks about serving God and others, and living a purposeful life, 'wherever' you might be. And I completely agree with that, to an extent. I say to an extent because I don't know that God's ideal plan for you is for you to work at any old job most of the week and then for you to try to get in the good stuff and make up for it on weekends. I don't think that is the best God can do in your life. I think He wants something better for His people.

I also say 'to an extent' because I sense that most people are using this 'serve wherever you are' argument more as a cop-out to keep from moving out in faith in their lives. Is the Holy Spirit leading you towards a different life's work? Let the term 'life's work' sink in a bit. Doesn't that give your career path a whole new meaning and level of importance?

I was in facilities management for 15 years, and I had another 20 years to go before reaching the age of normal, vocational retirement. The thought of spending the next 20 years of my life the same way I had spent the previous 15 years was discouraging to say the least. I shuddered to imagine myself at the age of 65 looking back and saying 'Is this what I did with my life?'

Is your 'life's work' crunching away at numbers in a cubicle for 40 years? It might be. I am not trying to tell anyone what God's leading and plan for their lives should or shouldn't be. I am just trying to encourage you to carefully consider the working of the Holy Spirit in your life, allowing Him to direct you to the purposeful life God has in store for you. As I mentioned already, I spent several decades as an expert at not following the leading of the Holy Spirit in my life, and I have the battle scars and regrets to prove it.

Are you an accountant while God is calling you to work with animals? Are you an executive in Corporate America while God is calling you to run a homeless shelter? Are you an electrician when God is calling you to be a doctor? Are you working in Corporate America when God is calling you to stay home with your children? Are you a mechanic when God is calling you to be a dentist? Are you a facilities manager when God is calling you to be a teacher and a writer (my example)? The sooner you answer the call of God on your life through the leading of the Holy Spirit, the sooner you will find purpose in your life, and the sooner you will be able to reach and maintain your ideal body weight.

I am a firm believer that a person is happy only to the extent they fulfill God's purpose for their life. But how can you know God's purpose for your life? You start with the known to find unknown. As an example, from reading this book, the known for you includes dietary holiness. Start there. You know you shouldn't be gossiping with your best friend every weekend. Start there. You know you shouldn't be looking at questionable things on the computer. Start there. You will find that God's purpose for your life begins to slowly unfold as the influences of the things of your flesh loosen their grip and your sensitivity to the things of the Spirit increase.

For those who are afraid of some unknown tragedy or pain that moving in the direction of the Holy Spirit's leading in your life might bring, consider these insightful words from Beth Moore.

'He (God) is determined to pursue you because He knows the greatest joy in your life will come from His plan for you.'

'We can live with all manner of tribulation more easily than we can live with purposelessness.'

'If you are to live out God's purpose for your life, you must come to a place where you determine a focus to your life.'

(*Discovering God's Purpose for Your Life*, pages 11, 12, and 16, respectively, by Beth Moore)

Your issue may not be your vocation. Your issue may be that God is calling you to teach a class or volunteer for service projects at your church and in your community. Your issue may be that, as a parent, the Holy Spirit is leading you to parent your children differently. But whatever the Holy Spirit is leading you to do, do it.

You will need to pursue purpose in your life in order to reach and maintain your ideal body weight. It is within the context of purposeful living that food addiction, and every other addiction, loses its appeal and grip on your life. When Satan can't lead you around by the nose with food addiction then he can't keep you from living your life at your ideal body weight.

It always feels so good to know we have defeated the enemy's power in our lives, to experience success in an area in which he once had us by the throat. I think it is a good practice for the Believer to celebrate and rejoice over the victories we experience as we walk in obedience to God's Word. Every time I watch a baptism, for example, I sing in my head 'And another one slips away from the enemy.'

God wants you to live a purposeful, meaningful, and abundant life. God wants to position you to do something awesome in your life. Stop living your life like the prodigal son, choosing to wallow in the mud with the pigs. God promises a meaningful and abundant life to those who live His way. It is Satan, the thief, who desires to steal that birthright from you. Living your life at your ideal body weight is your birthright as a Believer.

"The thief cometh not, but for to steal, and to kill, and to destroy: I am come that they might have life, and that they might have it more abundantly." (John 10:10, KJV)

Satan is that thief whose worldly wisdom and ways are designed to steal, kill, and destroy any chance of you living a meaningful, purpose-filled life. He is the one telling you that you are overweight because you are lazy and weak. He is the one telling you that you can treat your body any way you want. And Satan is the one that wants to tease you into the types of ungodly escapes that will only hinder your chances of reaching your ideal body weight.

Through Jesus Christ, you now have access to the power (or fruit) of the Holy Spirit in your life through spiritual conditioning. You need to draw upon that power to ensure a righteous motivation that will result in permanent weight loss. Satan is the great deceiver, whose worldly wisdom and ways will only lead you down a path to failure.

"For such are false apostles, deceitful workers, transforming themselves into apostles of Christ. And no wonder! For Satan himself transforms himself into an angel of light. Therefore it is no great thing if his ministers also transform themselves into ministers of righteousness, whose end will be according to their works." (II Corinthians 11:13-15, NKJV, BibleGateway.com)

Most have not received, or will not receive, the wisdom of God regarding weight loss. It is no wonder that the success rate is so low, with more and more people joining the ranks of the overweight each year. But you are on the right track. You will not be deceived by Satan's worldly wisdom. You will be among the few who find God's Weigh to your ideal body weight.

"Enter ye in at the strait gate: for wide is the gate, and broad is the way, that leadeth to destruction, and many there be which go in thereat: because strait is the gate, and narrow is the way, which leadeth unto life, and few there be that find it. Beware of false prophets, which come to you in sheep's clothing, but inwardly they are ravening wolves." (Matthew 7:13-15, KJV)

At some point in each of our lives, maybe part of the mid-life crisis for many, we finally begin to sense that we want our lives to matter – to make a difference – to have meaning. I believe God would have us reach this mindset much earlier than mid-life, but such is the tendency. Coming to the realization that the pursuit of purpose will create a better life for you than the pursuit of pleasure is important for you as you seek to control your diet and work towards your ideal body weight.

All this is not to say that a life of purpose has no pleasure. The pursuit of purpose will provide deep, lasting pleasure. The pursuit of pleasure will ensure you have neither. So choose today to live the better life.

Let's apply this to your dietary and health-related choices by way of examples…

+ A focus on living a life of purpose will lead you to eat a piece of fruit, while pursuing a life of pleasure will lead you to eat a donut.
+ A focus on living a life of purpose will lead you to being in bed by 10:00PM (nothing good happens after 10:00PM),

while pursuing a life of pleasure may have you up past midnight watching television.

+ A focus on living a life of purpose will draw you away from alcohol and tobacco, while pursuing a life of pleasure may lead you to abuse these substances.

With each of these examples, I hope you can see that focusing on living a life of purpose will lead you to do things that enable you to become healthy and reach your ideal body weight, while a meaningless life focused on the pursuit of pleasure will not satisfy, will ruin your health, and will keep you from reaching your ideal body weight.

Focusing on living a life of purpose will affect every decision you make in life; who you will spend time with, what career you will pursue, how you invest your free time, and yes, it will influence your dietary and health choices.

As you seek to live a life of purpose rather than a life of pleasure, and as that focus begins to change your perspective, motivation, and life for the better, you will begin to notice that seeking comfort from an unhealthy diet, alcohol, a high-paying but poorly chosen career, tobacco, and entertainment no longer attracts you or even gets your attention. You will become more and more aware that all good things come from God, not from the pleasures and escapes you might seek to experience.

"Every good gift and every perfect gift is from above..." (James 1:17, KJV)

"In the way of righteousness is life: and in the pathway thereof there is no death." (Proverbs 12:28, KJV)

You will find that you are more interested in making life choices that positively serve your life of purpose, rather than making life choices solely intended to provide an escape. You will no longer require such escapes. You will eat your vegetables. You will turn down those desserts.

The pursuit of purpose in your life is an essential exercise to achieving and maintaining your ideal body weight. You must choose between a life that will be lived with purpose and a life that will be lived in the pursuit of pleasure. You can't have both.

"A double-minded man is unstable in all his ways." (James 1:8, KJV)

There is a better life waiting for you than the one offered by soda, donuts, and gluttony. Once you begin living a purpose-driven life you may find, as I did, that taking time out to eat is actually annoying. Therein you have the flip-side of what this book is all about; now eating to nourish your body because it is not yours to ignore.

This change will be a strange and wonderful experience for those who have never known a life that was not centered around food. It is a great feeling and lifestyle when you come to the point where you can enjoy food, but it doesn't control you; when you don't structure your life around your next meal or snack. As a former glutton, the most depressing words ever spoken at a buffet were 'I am too full to eat anymore.'

As I, you may find that life becomes so exciting for you that you can barely fall asleep at night, anxious to get to the next day. And having to bother with eating just seems to keep you from more of the really good stuff that comes with living a purpose-driven life; food taking a backseat to what life has to offer.

"Commit they works unto the Lord, and thy thoughts shall be established." (Proverbs 16:3, KJV)

As you begin living a life with Godly purpose you may find that you need to exercise some caution over the excitement and joy you will experience. You see, in this country, we have developed a bad habit of celebrating the victories and joys in our lives by destroying our bodies with one unhealthy practice or another. This can come in the form of alcohol, drugs, late nights, or for us 'good Christians', gluttonous and unhealthy eating.

Even within the context of a victory or joy I experience from living a life with Godly purpose, my flesh can try to draw me into a celebratory mode that involves sin. Like most people in this country, I am just so accustomed to doing something bad to celebrate even the good things in my life; finishing a big project at work, completing this book, a successful day of yard-work, celebrating someone's birthday or marriage, or just simply finding myself with a few days of rest and vacation.

Satan would take no greater pleasure than being able to take you from joy to sin in this way. Unfortunately, Satan and our flesh never take a vacation. We must be vigilant, alert, and sober at all times.

"Be sober, be vigilant; because your adversary the devil, as a roaring lion, walketh about, seeking whom he may devour." (I Peter 5:8, KJV)

As I, you must learn to experience and enjoy life for what it is, and in the way or form God has provided. Resist the temptation to add more (sin) to a positive, Godly experience.

If you want to take back your birthright of living at your ideal body weight you must develop a passion for the things of God and come to the point where you can say 'God, I want to be all that You want me to be. I want to go where You want me to go. I want to do what You want me to do.'

You will have to wake up every morning and make the decision to pursue purpose over pleasure. This must be a commitment that you make, and a stand that you take, every day for the rest of your life. This will not be a one-time thing.

You will be glad you did. God has a better life to offer you than the one you can make for yourself. The pursuit of purpose will create a better life for you than the pursuit of pleasure. A purpose-filled life will be essential for you to reach and maintain your ideal body weight.

"For the Lord God is a sun and shield: the Lord will give grace and glory: no good thing will he withhold from them that walk uprightly. O Lord of hosts, blessed is the man that trusteth in thee." (Psalm 84:11-12, KJV)

"... they that seek the Lord shall not want any good thing." (Psalm 34:10, KJV)

"Delight thyself also in the Lord; and he shall give thee the desires of thine heart." (Psalm 37:7, KJV)

Pleasure boasts itself as the single best route to happiness, but only purpose can ensure such a destination.

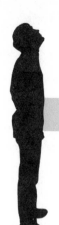
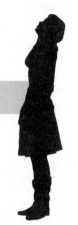

Chapter 9

A Righteous Motivation is Needed to Reach Your Ideal Body Weight

There are five spiritual keys to reaching your ideal body weight. They are recognition of ownership, spiritual conditioning, leading of the Holy Spirit, purposeful living, and righteous motivation.

God does not want you to be overweight, or any other Christian for that matter. The Christian community should be the healthiest and most attractive demographic on the face of the planet. The world should be beating a path to our door as they seek to learn of the secret that we must have regarding health and ideal body weight. In so doing, obedience to God regarding physical health could prove to be one of the greatest evangelical tools ever devised.

Just think, weight loss is the number one New Year's resolution year after year. The world obviously wants the secret. The world is looking for the secret. And God has the secret. But we have to look to God for it, apply it to our lives, and let the world see the results before anyone will knock on the door of our churches in an effort to understand how, why, and Who.

You are called to be a witness to the world by way of successful living. Seeking to be a good witness to the world of the wisdom and power of God in your life is an excellent and righteous motivation to reach your ideal body weight. Ideal body weight, as shallow as it may sound, is an area of successful living that will get the world's attention.

"For thou art an holy people unto the LORD thy God, and the LORD hath chosen thee to be a peculiar people unto himself, above all the nations that are upon the earth." (Deuteronomy 14:2, KJV)

The incorrect theology passed along in the Church today regarding passages like this is that God wanted His people to be peculiar by way of the things His people did, as if God gave His people a list of strange things to do that had no purpose other than getting the heathen nations' attention. Nothing could be more inaccurate.

If God only wanted Believers to get the world's attention by doing strange things without purpose, He could have simply mandated that all Christians wear pink shirts with purple polka-dots, and green hats. I think that would be more than sufficient to get the world's attention, differentiating us from the rest of the world as 'peculiar' for sure.

The point here is that God's directives and practices regarding Christian living will produce positive results in our lives that get the world's attention, not odd behavior. Peculiar means that the success Christian people should be experiencing in their lives (ideal body weight included) through the application of God's wisdom will leave the world bewildered and looking to us for help. Herein is one of God's purposes for your life, a righteous motivation to reach your ideal body weight, is to be a testimony to 'all the nations' of the wisdom and power of God in your life.

Walking out the Christian life will always do more to reach others for Christ than talk alone. I believe that few things create a greater contradiction in the minds of the world than overweight and unhealthy Christians. I know that sounds harsh, but in today's world of superficial and shallow focuses, I believe it to be an accurate statement.

We talk about the wisdom and power of God, but when the world sees that we are unable to control our diets and maintain our ideal body weight, there is a discrepancy in their minds between what we say and what they see. But on the flip-side, this also presents the Christian community with a great opportunity to reach the world for Christ.

And that is exactly what you are called to do, draw attention to all things God (to God). This is a righteous motivation. Here we have another component of God's will for your life, yet another component of God's will that will be part of reaching your ideal body weight and help lead you to purposeful living.

"What? Know ye not that your body is the temple of the Holy Ghost which is in you, which ye have of God, and ye are not your own? For ye are brought with a price: therefore glorify God in your body, and in your spirit, which are God's." (I Corinthians 6:19-20, KJV)

You are called to glorify God. The positive results that come about through obedience to God's Word are an essential part of how you do that. Glorifying God simply means that you are to conduct yourself in such a way that your actions and your speech (and corresponding life results like reaching your ideal body weight) draw positive attention to Him.

Understanding that your body is not your own, but God's, is another important way to ensure you have a proper (righteous) motivation for reaching your ideal body weight. We talked extensively about this in an earlier chapter.

It is in understanding and acknowledging that your body is not your own that you will find the motivation that sustains you. Even during those times when you have no concern for your health and body weight, understanding that your body is not yours to abuse will keep you on track to reaching and maintaining your ideal body weight.

In contrast to righteous motivations, there are fleshly, unrighteous motivations for reaching your ideal body weight. For example, your motivation might be to fit into a revealing bathing suit or tight clothing. This motivation defies every principle and desire of God regarding living a Godly, modest life. God certainly doesn't want you drawing others into lust. That is not His will for your life.

An unrighteous motivation will have a degenerative effect on the spiritual conditioning so needed to walk obediently with regard to dietary holiness. Don't believe Satan's lie that the more motivations, of any kind, the better. The source of your motivation, if not Godly, may be the very thing that sabotages your journey towards reaching your ideal body weight. Trying to find motivation for weight loss in fleshly things does not produce a purpose-driven, successful, Godly life. This is not a righteous motivation.

"For he that soweth to his flesh shall of the flesh reap corruption but he that soweth to the Spirit shall of the Spirit reap life everlasting." (Galatians 6:8, KJV)

"… Walk in the Spirit, and ye shall not fulfill the lust of the flesh. For the flesh lusteth against the Spirit, and the Spirit against the flesh: and these are contrary the one to the other: so that yet cannot do the things that ye would. But if ye be led of the Spirit, ye are not under the law. Now the works of the flesh are manifest, which are these; adultery, fornication, uncleanness, lasciviousness, idolatry, witchcraft, hatred, varience, emulations, wrath, strife, seditions, heresies, envyings, murders, drunkenness, revellings, and such like of which I tell you in time past, that they which do such things shall not inherit the kingdom of God. But the fruit of the Spirit is love, joy, peace, longsuffering, gentleness, goodness, faith, meekness, temperance: against such things there is no law. And they that are Christ's have crucified the flesh with the affections and lusts. If we live in the Spirit, let us also walk in the Spirit. Let us not be desirous of vain glory, provoking one another, envying one another." (Galatians 5:16-26, KJV)

The motivations of the flesh to reach your ideal body weight, and working to entice the flesh of others for that matter, will ensure you never have the spiritual strength to get there, or at the very least, that you will still be miserable and unsatisfied even if you do. Fleshly motivations will not produce purposeful living in your life. And you will need peace, longsuffering (patience), and temperance (self-control) in order to reach your ideal body weight in a Godly, lasting manner.

Prayer is another important component of successful living. Prayer is part of a life lived with purpose and is essential to spiritual conditioning. And prayer is essential to reaching your ideal body weight. But unfortunately, a vain, ungodly motivation for reaching your ideal body weight will ensure God will not be inclined to bless you in this way. Although it is God's will for your life that you live your life at your ideal body weight, it is not God's will for your life that you look great so you can use your body to fulfill the lusts of your flesh and cause someone else to do the same.

"… ye have not , because ye ask not. Ye ask, and receive not, because you ask amiss, that ye may consume it upon your lusts… God resisteth the proud, but giveth grace unto the humble." (James 4:2,3,6, KJV)

So if your motivation for losing weight is out of pride and vanity then you will not have God partnering with you to reach your goal. Your prayers to God to enable you to reach your ideal body weight will not be acceptable, because you ask amiss, that you might consume this blessing upon your lustful nature. This is no small statement.

Now this is not to say that you will not experience great pleasure in living a life at your ideal body weight. It's just the sinful pleasures that need to be avoided. There will be plenty of pleasure. I hope I haven't led you to believe that the life ahead of you will be some sufferable existence. That is not the case at all.

It is a great pleasure to feel in sync with the will of God for your life and to experience the working of God's wisdom in your life; growing in faith regarding His ways. It is a great pleasure to experience physical vitality for living and to be able to perform at very high levels at work, play, and home due to improved health. It is a great pleasure to buy clothing that fits well and to be able to sit, move, bend, and get about comfortably. It is a great pleasure to not be controlled by the lusts of the flesh and this world, and to know that you are a positive witness to others.

It is a great pleasure to teach others the same Godly wisdom that has brought you to your ideal body weight. It is a great pleasure knowing that you have set aside yet another stumbling block between you and experiencing God's best for your life. It is a great pleasure to be physically attracted to your spouse, and vice-versa. It is a great pleasure to experience all that life has to offer without the distraction and control of unhealthy living.

Consider those who are motivated to stay fit because they want to be attractive to the opposite sex. Is this a good long-term motivation? Just ask anyone who has been married more than a few months. If the motivation to stay fit for you is only for this reason, the difference between your wedding photo and your 10-year anniversary photo will have others wondering if they are even of the same person.

Your motivation to stay fit can go out the door in about as little time as it takes to say 'I do,' maybe long enough to last until the ice sculpture at your wedding reception has melted if you are lucky. God's Weigh will sustain. Man's ways will crumble and melt under the pressures of real life.

I think most would agree that God is a 'god of the heart.' While our actions, and even the apparent good results, may seem of God, He is primarily concerned about the condition of our hearts, our motivation, if you will.

"... the Lord seeth not as man seeth; for man looketh on the outward appearance, but the Lord looketh on the heart." (Samuel 16:7, KJV)

This is not to say that God is not concerned about you living your life at your ideal body weight, because He is. God is interested in both your heart and your actions. But God wants good things in your life to come about by way of a pure heart.

God does not want us to be like the Pharisees, whose motivation for observing the traditions of the elders was all for show, although they presented their actions as their attempt to honor God. Let's not pretend we are trying to honor God by walking in the truths outlined in this book, when our motivation is fleshly. You have to do this God's Weigh, not man's way.

"There is a way which seemeth right unto a man, but the end thereof are the ways of death." (Proverbs 14:12, KJV)

Success and failure can come in many different packages. Certainly, allowing our bodies to degenerate into an ill and overweight condition certainly constitutes failure. But does someone with a very healthy body represent success? Not necessarily. It depends on their heart towards God.

I would contend that if this healthy person was only motivated to stay fit because of the praise and adoration they receive from others, and/or an attempt to mask their personal weaknesses by way of a good appearance, that person has failed. Their 'success' is nothing more than another addiction.

So when I note that a fleshy motivation will not lead to success, keep in mind that the outward appearance of some may 'seem' to present a contradiction to that claim. But that is not the case. Remember, God looks at the heart, not the outward appearance. The heart should be our focus of concern as well.

Not only does appealing to one's flesh for motivation not work, but God explicitly prohibits such in His Word.

"... make no provision for the flesh, to fulfill the lusts thereof." (Romans 13:14, KJV)

That is a direct command, the violation of which constitutes sin. And we know full well that sin leads to death, or in this case, death to your journey to your ideal body weight in a Godly, sustainable way.

"Then when lust hath conceived, it bringeth forth sin: and sin, when it is finished, bringeth forth death." (James 1:15, KJV)

There are those who seem to have been able to successfully adhere to a fit lifestyle for many years without one conscious thought of God and His ways. So what about them? Their death is primarily spiritual and emotional. These individuals have sowed to their flesh so much and so often that it is controlling them completely. And I emphasize that their flesh is controlling them.

A righteous motivation is important to achieving your ideal body weight in a Godly, sustainable way; ensuring that through it all you will be whole in spirit, soul, and body. Desiring to be a witness to the world of the wisdom and power of God, and acknowledging that it is your responsibility to care for your body on God's behalf, are two righteous motivations that will help you reach and maintain your ideal body weight.

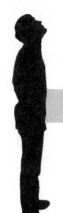
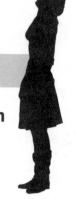

Chapter 10

Man's Wisdom Verses God's Wisdom

I would think that a large room (maybe multiple large rooms) could be filled from top to bottom, front to back, and side to side with all the books, magazines, articles, and e-mails that have been written on diet and weight loss. And 99+% of that material would be man's wisdom, one angle or viewpoint after another regarding how to reach your ideal body weight, each contradicting the other.

This material would include a lot of technical viewpoints and philosophies regarding diet and weight loss, with little material regarding any healthy or righteous motivations for following through with the technical information. Some of the technical information might be good. But then there would be a large amount that would be bad. And you wouldn't be able to separate the good from the bad without embarking on a life-long process of using yourself as a guinea-pig as you test each theory. God warns us that you should expect this kind of 'foolishness' if we seek man for wisdom and not Him; if we fail to seek God's Weigh.

"... the wisdom of this world is foolishness with God..." (I Corinthians 3:19, KJV)

So there you would be, with a mountain of material to study through. And what would you get for all your study and application time? You would approach each diet with a worldly motivation for success for starters, guaranteeing failure due to a lack of spiritual support required, regardless of how good the technical information might be.

And as you try method after method, viewpoint after viewpoint, over the next twenty to thirty years of your life, you may seem to show progress with some of the methods, at least for a short time. But with each you slip off into unhealthy eating again, gaining all of the weight you lost on their programs, and some more atop all of that.

There is a reason why you tend to gain more weight back after ending a diet and exercise program than you lost during it. This happens because the chemical and hormonal condition these programs create in your body makes your body more of a fat-storing machine than it was before you began. And this occurs because most diet and exercise plans attempt to force your body to lose weight.

You can't force your body to breathe less (for long) and you can't force your body to lose weight long-term. God created our bodies, and man's wisdom will not force it to do anything in a successful and sustainable fashion. Eventually, the change in the chemical and hormonal condition in your body, as it attempts to correct the imbalances the diet produced through lack of nutrients and the burnout caused by the intense exercise program, leaves you with food cravings and fatigue that cannot be resisted. So you fall off the plan, left with a body more susceptible to gaining weight than before. So much for all of your time, effort, and money.

I think there is also a psychological/emotional re-coil effect that not only leaves a person in a fat-storing mode physically, but it leaves a person in an emotional condition (failure and depression) that results in less control (willpower) over their diets than they had before starting the program.

Many of the techniques (gimmicks) being promoted out there are trying to make the body get into some chemically, hormonally advantageous orientation for weight loss. This is actually the correct approach, but it has to be done God's Weigh. At least someone has stumbled across something good after 50 years of error; some acknowledgement that the body is intelligently designed. But then the attempt made is to trick the body into working in ways that God never designed for it to work (error in man's calculations and conclusions).

Gimmick programs include everything from the low-carb diet to the ice-cream diet (yes there actually was one) to the grapefruit diet to the low-fat diet to a vegetarian diet to exercise programs that will cause you to shed the pounds or die trying. And those exercise programs are all about you becoming obsessed with your body. This is not God's Weigh.

Weight loss is also approached by some with the belief that the body acts in a linear fashion; calories in verses calories out. Nothing could be further from the truth. God designed your body with the greatest of intelligence; designed to protect you.

Try to overly restrict calories and your body will slow down its metabolism to conserve nutrients and energy. Try to exercise excessively and your body will again slow down its metabolism to conserve nutrients and energy. Try to consume loads of coffee to get you into a supposed hyper weight loss condition and your body will experience uncontrollable hunger cravings for all the nutrients and energy used up from the chemically-induced emergency responses that caffeine causes in the body.

God designed the body to always seek balance; equilibrium. Hold your breath for one minute and your body will then force you to breath in even more air during the second minute than you would have over the same two minutes of normal breathing. You can't fight that. God's dietary plan will not kick your body into this type of equilibrium balancing, over-compensating process that leads to fat-storage. God's dietary plan will keep you in equilibrium at all times; avoiding the over-compensation that results in weight gain, and even in degenerative diseases over time.

You should be aware that even now, as you are about to embark on a diet plan that pleases God, your body is most likely chemically, hormonally, and nutritionally out of equilibrium. Your body may be in fat-storage mode. What does this mean to you? It means that you could literally gain a few pounds of fat initially as you work with your body to supply the nutrients it needs, and as you wait for your body to right itself chemically and hormonally from the abuses it has undergone up until this point.

In all likelihood you may not see a gain on the scales itself. But this will be mainly because the water loss you experience over the first several weeks will more than compensate for any possible fat-storage. So you should still expect to experience a net loss on the scales over those first few weeks.

On man's diet plans, everyone expects and experiences weight loss quickly and somewhat easily on the front-end. This is then followed by weeks of ever-decelerating weight loss, and eventually for many, even a complete stagnation in progress. All the while, the difficulty of staying with the diet plan just keeps getting harder and harder as well. This is not God's Weigh.

This is why most weight loss testimonials are based on the results clients have exerienced in the first few weeks only. And of course, this first few weeks is when the most water weight is lost as well. The slowed mebolism from their restrictive diets has not yet set in.

As you approach weight loss and getting healthy God's Weigh, your body's equilibrium and strength will improve with each passing week. As the health of your body and its supply of nutrients increases over time, your food/nutrient cravings will decrease. With the exception of those first two or three weeks of water loss, you may very well find that you lose weight/fat more and more quickly with each passing week.

In any event, you may want to consider not weighing yourself at all. The fitness world says weighing yourself regularly is an important key to sticking with a weight loss program. It might be if you are trying to reach your ideal body weight man's way and not God's Weigh. That is man's wisdom, not God's wisdom. And along these same lines, don't measure yourself either.

Keeping focused on your weight loss progress (or weight gain if underweight) can have the effect of working more with your flesh than with the Spirit. And it's the things of the Spirit that produce life (success) in our lives, while the things of the flesh produce death (failure) in our lives. Keep your focus on successfully walking in obedience to God's dietary directives. Don't focus on the results.

It isn't good to get overly focused on the weight loss, especially initially. What matters is that you follow God's dietary directives and gain good health. Man's wisdom says that you need to lose weight before you can be healthy. God's Weigh says that you need to be healthy before you can lose weight.

I would also encourage you to not even look at your body in the mirror, at least not without clothes on, and not even then whenever possible. You might think that this is impossible, but it isn't. It just takes a little practice and ingenuity at times. I find this practice to be extremely helpful in keeping me from developing a fleshly motivation and mindset regarding the appearance of my body.

I find I can get knocked off course when I allow myself to become too mindful of my body be weighing it or seeing it in the mirror. If your strength is coming from the Spirit and not the flesh, these fleshly sources of motivation will actually work against you in the long-run.

Along these same lines, even if you are 100+ pounds overweight, you need to be content with where you are right now. I know that sounds strange. But the most important thing that you can experience through this process is learning to walk in obedience to God, almost ignoring the positive results that are sure to come. Freedom from Satan's grip on your life and dietary choices is the greatest victory here; reaching your ideal body weight being icing on the cake (pardon the expression).

All of this, and everything you find in this book, applies to those suffering with anorexia and bulimia as well. Reaching your ideal body weight, whether by losing weight or gaining weight, is all about walking in obedience to God's Word regarding diet and health. It applies to the overweight, to the underweight, and to the unhealthy moderate-weight.

You are completely loved by God right now, just as you are. He is just happy that you are now turning to Him, gladly receiving you as the father of the prodigal son. God is not concerned that it will take some time for the spiritual growth you have experienced to show up in weight loss and achieving your ideal body weight. The victory is already yours. In that you can relax and be patient concerning your weight loss journey.

Let obedience to God's Word be your primary objective, losing those extra pounds being a secondary benefit. This mindset (a highly spiritually conditioned mindset) will do wonders towards keeping you patient and feeding the things of the Spirit (life) over the things of the flesh (death). You will find this to be a very freeing approach. You are on a spiritual journey even more than you are on a physical journey, although the results for both will be positive.

Believe it or not, your excess body weight is your body's attempt to protect itself. For example, toxic build-up in the body will cause the body to store fat as a means of creating a buffer between the toxins and your internal organs.

Your body will always respond to a particular order of priority when it comes to protecting itself, and unfortunately, it usually isn't in a direction that is favorable to your appearance. Your body will seek to protect its internal organs and general health by redirecting nutrients from your hair follicles if necessary (hair loss), by accumulating fat within which to store toxins (wider waistline), by trying to conserve energy through a slowed metabolism (fatigue and fat gain throughout the body), and/or by redirecting alkalizing nutrients from your teeth to balance your blood chemistry (tooth decay and loss).

The type of fat formed in the event of toxic build-up is called visceral fat. Unlike what we think of as normal, 'flabby' fat (or subcutaneous fat) that forms just beneath the surface of the skin, this fat forms inside the midsection musculature (cavity) of your body, in and around your internal organs.

Visceral fat is the type of fat that can make a man look like he is 9-months pregnant; sometimes even men who are otherwise thin elsewhere on their bodies. If you were to thump their stomachs it would be like thumping a watermelon; strangely firm. This is because the visceral fat is under the midsection musculature, not between the midsection musculature and the skin. We typically are thinking of subcutaneous fat when we think of fat; the soft, malleable, flabby, and eventually sagging type that forms just under the skin on our legs, arms, chest, rear, face, back, outside our midsection, etc.

Health 'experts' contend that visceral fat is the most dangerous kind of fat. That is not an accurate statement. An accurate statement is that the body is in a dangerous state of ill-health, trying to protect itself from an excessive build-up of toxins through the accumulation of toxin-storing visceral fat.

The danger component in all this is that the body is in a very poor state of health. The visceral fat is a safety mechanism designed to protect your internal organs to the best of its ability. What the visceral fat does provide is a warning that the body has reached a very unhealthy, degenerative condition.

Excess water retention operates by the same type of protective principle; accumulating water throughout the body as necessary to protect its cells from the excessive toxins present. The loss of 'bloat' from the release of this excess water from your body will be the earliest indication that you are heading down a healthy path.

So we need to work in harmony with how God designed our bodies, and this can only happen as we follow His directives concerning diet. And the nice thing is, for those of you who don't care a lick about the science of the body, you don't need to know anything about how the body works to reach your ideal body weight. Just obey God. He never intended for anyone to hurt their brains with all that information.

"… of making many books there is no end; and much study is a weariness of the flesh. Let us hear the conclusion of the whole matter: Fear God, and keep his commandments; for this is the whole duty of man." (Ecclesiastes 12:12-13, KJV)

Please get this firmly into your thinking. Man will never fully understand the human body; at least not enough to make it do and perform as desired through some clever trick or angle on diet. The world, and the Church unfortunately, has been waiting for man to make that breakthrough in science (find that trick / magic pill) for the past 50 years, and longer.

Stop looking to the world for the solution. Stop being so kind and patient with the world's chronic series of mistakes and failures. There is no need for you to volunteer to be part of their science experiment any longer.

"It is better to trust in the Lord than to put confidence in man." (Psalm 118:8, KJV)

God is not about the confusion and failure you will find in this room of fitness material. God is about clarity and success. Satan is the author of the confusion and failure that you find in this man-made fitness collection.

"… God is not the author of confusion, but of peace…" (I Corinthians 14:33, KJV)

"The way of the wicked is as darkness: they know not at what they stumble." (Proverbs 4:19, KJV)

And then possibly after twenty to thirty years of trial and failure, you finally decide being overweight is just the way you were meant to be. You have bought into Satan's lie. And besides, now, after all those years, you figure you are too old to worry with all that anyway (maybe a reflection that your motivation was flesh-based to begin with).

You concede that you will simply join the ranks of the rest of the ever-widening 40-somethings, 50-somethings, and 60-somethings (not to mention kids, teenagers, 20-somethings and 30-somethings these days). Satan has successfully deceived you and worked his way and will in yet another person's life. Satan has added another notch of success in his quest to keep God's people tired, sick, and overweight.

And if you are like most, throughout that entire time, you would have never looked to God's Word for the solution to your struggle with body weight. You either just didn't know it was in there or you might have been afraid to find out what God had to say on the subject.

Perhaps you have attended a weight loss program at a local church along the way, but the program/book selected was written with the wisdom of the world. Unfortunately, ungodly, man-made wisdom, even if studied within the sanctity of a church building, still results in ungodly, man-made results.

Another issue with that large room full of dietary and weight loss materials is all the reading time it would take to get through it all, even if you could find it all and afford it all. Shouldn't we expect God to have a more efficient way of communicating most of that same information; all of which we could trust as accurate and beneficial at that? Well, He has provided just that in the Bible.

Based on the fact that you are reading this book now, you have determined that maybe God does have something to say about your health and body weight, which is a breakthrough in and of itself. You have set fear aside to come see what God wants to say to you about your health and body weight, yet another breakthrough. You are on your way to victory. I am happy to report that you will not be adding to any overweight statistics anymore. And I will be singing 'And another one slips away from the enemy.'

This book is about equipping you to overcome the works and deceptions of Satan in your life, taking back what is yours. As a Believer, living at your ideal body weight is your birthright. Get righteously angry and determined if you have to. Don't let Satan and man's wisdom keep you from your birthright any longer.

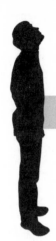
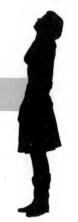

Chapter 11

Lifespan: Evidence of a Problem

The predominance of overweight and unhealthy people in this country is a reality that has reached epidemic proportions that exceed any plague found in Scripture; second only to the world flood in total damage. That is no small statement. That should be more than enough to prove to you that something is wrong; that Godly wisdom is missing from the equation.

Poor health and excess weight should be enough to show you that the Church is far from understanding, accepting, and applying Biblical truth regarding diet and health in the Christian community. The Church is denying the very power and wisdom of God needed for each Believer to reach their ideal body weight and good health, looking rather to the world and its man-made wisdom and recommendations on the subject. That is such a tragedy. The world should be looking to us for the solution to reaching one's ideal body weight and obtaining good health, in all matters as far as that goes.

I want you to now see yet another very revealing truth that highlights our deviation from God's ways regarding diet and health. It is with respect to the topic of lifespan. More specifically, it is with respect to the incredible discrepancy between how long the average person lives in this country and how long God says we should be living.

A quick disclaimer – I realize that pollution and other factors largely beyond our individual control can negatively affect our lifespans. I know that the quality of the foods available to most of us is often questionable. We can't forget about the inoculations given to us as children that may have had long-term negative effects on our health and lifespans either. And as I mentioned earlier, unforgiveness and bitterness can negatively affect your physical health as significantly as a poor diet, alcohol, and tobacco.

In order to make progress in taking back the lost potential due to factors beyond our control in the immediate term, the Christian community will need to lead a revolution in this country and around the world against industries and governmental powers whose ungodly activities negatively affect our physical well-being.

Further discussion of such a revolution is certainly beyond the scope of this book. I mainly wanted to highlight that I realize that there are factors negatively affecting your health and lifespan over which you had and/or have no control.

But I think we should be able to agree or expect that we can significantly bridge the gap between how long God says we should be living and how long we are actually living by way of obedience to the things God's Word directs us to do that we can control. The Church demographic should have a noticeably longer lifespan than the rest of the world, but we don't. Why? Because we have not sought and applied Godly wisdom to the issue of health, ideal body weight, and lifespan. It is as simple as that.

Are we living as long as God intended? Most would argue that we are doing great. The average lifespan in this country is at an all-time high so the statistics say; the upper 70's. We must be doing something right, so we think.

As with all things, and as encouraged in Proverbs 3:5-8, let's not spend too much time 'leaning on our own understanding.' But rather let's look to God for the measure of our success in this regard.

"Trust in the LORD *with all your heart, and lean not on your own understanding. In all your ways acknowledge Him, and He shall direct your*

paths. Do not be wise in your own eyes. Fear the LORD *and depart from evil. It will be health to your flesh and strength to your bones." (Proverbs 3:5-8, NKJV, BibleGateway.com)*

Are you surprised to hear that God's Word tells us how long we should live? Would you be surprised to hear that God's Word also tells us how long a sinful people live? Would you then be surprised to learn that our lifespans equal those of the sinful people that God references in the Bible? If so, you will be in for many more surprises throughout the remainder of this book as you see that God speaks very directly to your dietary practices and health. So what is God's standard for lifespan and how do we measure up?

Prior to the introduction of man's sin into the world, the lifespan of mankind was infinite. As the Biblical record would indicate, after man's fall into sin, lifespans were certainly not infinite, but did reach into the upper 900's. I tend to believe that the necessity that God allow degeneration in our bodies (aging) came about because of the need for a process of sanctification in our lives due to the introduction of sin into the world.

And then, mankind went from sin to what might be termed 'mass sin', to which God responded by declaring that the lifespan of man would be shortened to 120 years. This is the last time God made a declaration regarding what our lifespans 'should be.'

"... man... his days shall be an hundred and twenty years." (Genesis 6:3, KJV)

It is important to note that God did not zap this declared lifespan into immediate reality. As is often the case, God used His creation to accomplish His/this declaration over time. God is not as often a zapper-god as most would contend, again, working more often through His creation. Those who were over 120 years of age did not suddenly drop dead. Noah was several hundred years beyond this mark when he exited the ark, and lived several hundred years longer.

So how did God bring about his 120 year declaration? The Genesis 6:3 declaration was made before the world flood. It was through the world flood that God achieved this declaration. As we study the Biblical record we can see that many generations came and went before the lifespan of man ultimately reduced down from the 900's to 120.

The original design of the Earth included a water canopy in the upper atmosphere (Genesis 1:6-7). To accomplish the massive flood God used waters from within the earth and waters from above the earth (the water canopy). With an elimination or reduction in the water canopy as a result of its disintegration into rain, as we might imagine, there were changes in atmospheric pressure, the electromagnetic field, oxygen level, and radiation on the Earth's surface, all to the detriment of our bodies.

This reality is further supported by the fact that the decline in lifespan from the 900's to 120 over time, when graphed, forms a reverse exponential curve. You may not know what an exponential curve is; however, any scientist or engineer will tell you that the exponential curve is one of the most basic and fundamental models of how the Earth functions.

More specifically, natural decline/decay/degeneration in nature follows a reverse exponential curve, which substantially supports that the reduction in lifespan over time occurred due to the degenerative affect the world flood process had on our environment.

So now we have God's standard for our lifespan, 120 years. But we are not living anywhere close to that. As a matter of fact, we are living only about two-thirds as long as that; 80 years at best on the average. And to make it even worse, at least the last 30 years of that 80-year life, for most of us, is spent struggling with various degenerative health issues and body weight problems.

We must be doing something wrong. We must be void in Godly wisdom to account for such a discrepancy between God's standard for our lifespan and the lifespan we are actually experiencing. God decided to go ahead and make it perfectly clear to us in Psalm 90 what the problem is, at least for those who want to know His truth on the matter.

For you to reach your ideal body weight God's Weigh, you will have to be one of those people who wants to know God's truth, regardless of how uncomfortable it may make you. You must be fearless in seeking out the truth of God's Word on any life issue. Relative to health and ideal body weight, the Church, as a whole, has been too afraid. The Church has shown that 'it can't handle the truth.'

"For we have been consumed by Your anger, and by Your wrath we are terrified. You have set our iniquities before You, our secret sins in the light of Your countenance. For all our days have passed away in Your wrath. We finish our years like a sigh. The days of our lives are seventy years; and if by reason of strength they are eighty years, yet their boast is only labor and sorrow; for it is soon cut off, and we fly away. Who knows the power of Your anger? For as the fear of You, so is Your wrath. So teach us to number our days, that we may gain a heart of wisdom." (Psalm 90:7-12, NKJV, BibleGateway.com)

Read through and meditate over this passage several times. There is a lot to unpack here. I have underlined the segments that I will expand upon next.

'we have been consumed' – I believe this to be a reference to poor health, degenerative disease, and loss of physical vitality in general.

'by Your anger, and by Your wrath' – Oftentimes, when the Bible refers to God's wrath, it does not mean that God is firing lightning bolts of turmoil into our lives. God's wrath is simply the natural negative consequences of violating His creation/system and life-principles for living. We have been consumed by God's wrath in that we are experiencing the negative consequences of ungodly living. This points to the fact that it is a 'sinful people' who only live 70 to 80 years.

'our secret sins' – I can't think of any more secret of a sin in the Church today than that of unhealthy eating. And the way the Church is able to pull it off, so to speak, is by denying that God has a holy standard that applies to the way we eat to begin with. We have even worked to misinterpret Scripture in order to satisfy our fleshly lust. That is what makes it such a 'secret sin'. It is no wonder that the Church doesn't want the truth. It is no wonder the Church is tired, sick, overweight, and living only a fraction of the years God intended.

'we finish our years like a sigh' – I have also seen 'like a sigh' shown as 'with a whimper'. Isn't this exactly what we are seeing today? It is bad enough that we are only living two-thirds as long as we should. But on top of that we live out those final 30 years with a whimper; in a state of obesity, fatigue, and degenerative disease. So not only are we shorting ourselves (and God and others) by 40 years, but then the years that we do have are lived out in poor health.

'The days of our lives are seventy years; and if by reason of strength they are eighty years' – This pretty much nails our 75+/- average lifespan in this country. This text tells us that God is talking about us, the current Church, in this passage. It's interesting that Moses wrote Psalm 90. He lived to 120. So the 'theoretical' 120-year lifespan and the 'sinful' 70-year to 80-year lifespan was a reality and discrepancy that existed way back in Moses' day. It also supports the argument that a significantly improved average lifespan is possible for God's people today.

'teach us to number our days, that we may gain a heart of wisdom' – This directive is exactly what I am doing here via a discussion of lifespan. If we number our days (70 to 80 years) and compare them with God's standard for our lifespan (120 years), then we can be open to God's wisdom/solution so that 'we may gain a heart of wisdom.'

We are living our lives, in many respects, no differently than the world around us. And we are consequently not living any longer than they. We are too busy looking to their ways when they should be looking to us and God's Weigh.

God's people are lost in a world of deception, darkness, and denial relative to God's principles for living a healthy life. The Christian community has absolutely refused to acknowledge that God has provided us with the dietary instructions required to be a healthy people. And we have denied that those instructions are commandments, calling for our obedience. Consequently, it is no wonder that we are as tired, sick, and overweight as we have become; living only a fraction of the life God intended.

We have made a mockery of the day-to-day value of our faith in front of a world that is looking for life answers, as we stumble in the same darkness as they, in search of a magic pill to restore us to health. In our actions and beliefs, we communicate to the world that God does not have the answers to life's important questions. We have communicated that God's ways are not sufficient to meet all our needs.

We especially make a mockery of God's Word when we pray for good health, all the while drinking sodas and eating donuts. Don't pray for health. Obey for health. This is not to discount the value of prayer. But to pray for God to heal someone's lung cancer while they continue to smoke three packs of cigarettes a day is a foolish mockery of God.

"Fools make a mock at sin…" (Proverbs 14:9, KJV)

"… be sure your sins will find you out." (Numbers 32:23, KJV)

"Be not deceived; God is not mocked; for whatsoever a man soweth, that shall he also reap." (Galatians 6:7, KJV)

I think by now you can see that we have a problem, whether we look at quality of life or quantity of life, and as we consider our poor witness to the world. The evidence of the problem is overwhelming.

Some might try to argue that we will each die when God wants us to die; meaning that no matter how we live our lives it will not impact our lifespan. One only needs to look as far as the topic of suicide to discount this myth. No one who has committed suicide has died on the day that God had willed for them. An unhealthy, ungodly diet is nothing more than slow suicide. So yes, your departure from God's ways will, in fact, negatively affect your lifespan, and the quality of your life to boot. Sin will always work against God's will and best for your life, lifespan included.

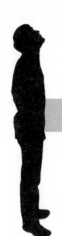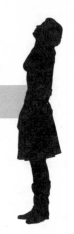

Chapter 12

How Did We Get This Way To Start With?

How did we manage to get ourselves into such a physical mess anyway? It's not like we wake up one day suddenly 50+ pounds overweight, with diabetes. It is because one day after another we choose to live each day apart from God's wisdom and power. That is why we are overweight. And the solution to reaching your ideal body weight is, one day after another moving forward, seeking God's wisdom and power on the subject of diet and health.

Why are we humans so prone to such neglect? In many cases I think it is because we think that we will somehow end up in a different place than everyone else who has traveled the same path; that we will somehow not be overweight and dealing with degenerative conditions like most everyone else over 40 years of age. Although the days may seem long the years pass by so quickly, and we wake up twenty years later looking and feeling like everyone else. Maybe there is a tendency in each of us, or better said a common deception of Satan in our lives, to think we will somehow defy the odds and not be subject to the same life principles and consequences as others.

I can recall having that mindset when I broke my arm at the age of twelve. The doctor told me that it would take six weeks for the bone to heal. Going into the three-week checkup, despite what the doctor had said, I thought I would be different from the norm. I was hopeful that he would see that my arm had already healed up and that my cast would be coming right off. I was wrong. I was just like everyone else. I had to go the full six weeks before I could get that annoying cast off.

The best thing for you to do is to expect to travel down the same path and reach the same undesired destination as those who have lived the same life you are living. You know that is not where you want to go. Stop living in a state of denial that says you will meet with a different end than they.

To expect otherwise, to not learn from the error of those who have gone before, is unwise. After all, isn't insanity the belief that you can keep on doing the same things over and over again while expecting different results, or that you can live the same life as someone else and end up in a better place than they?

We just don't want to think about the long-term consequences of our sinful choices. That is Satan's plan; his method for ensuring that we wake up twenty to thirty years down the road astonished and disappointed with where we have ended up. God warned us that this would be our tendency.

"Because sentence against an evil work is not executed speedily, therefore the heart of the sons of men is fully set in them to do evil." (Ecclesiastes 8:11, KJV)

Nowhere is the truth of Ecclesiastes 8:11 played out more precisely and dramatically than in the area of physical health. As youth or young adults, we openly and freely subject our bodies to abuses as if the 'day of consequence' will never come. Typically, it's only when we begin hitting our 40's and 50's that the decline in our physical, mental, and emotional vitality begins to get our attention.

The thing we dislike first, and possibly the most, is the excess weight we have gained. We find our energy levels declining with each passing year. We then begin to experience degenerative conditions like diabetes, arthritis, digestive disorders, and other unwelcome conditions.

Ultimately, we find ourselves struggling with life-threatening physical ailments that may be beyond repair or reversal.

God doesn't want us to experience this in our lives. God's plan is that we carefully consider the consequences that our sinful choices will ultimately bring about in our lives early in life, before the damage is done.

"Remember now thy Creator in the days of thy youth, while the evil days come not, nor the years draw nigh, when thou shalt say, I have no pleasure in them." *(Ecclesiastes 12:1, KJV)*

The actual Hebrew word translated 'while' here, which implies what comes after is inevitable (years of no pleasure), is a poor translation. The more accurate translation is 'so that.' So this is pointing to the importance of remembering God and His ways 'so that' you will not meet with years within which you have no pleasure.

You may already be in the midst of those years. I see 50-year olds, 40-year olds, and even 30-year olds and younger, who are already in the midst of those pleasure-less years. But remember that God is longsuffering towards you. By beginning again to 'remember thy Creator,' living in obedience to His Word, you can once again regain the mental, emotional, and physical health needed to experience years of pleasure.

"The Lord is not slack concerning his promise, as some men count slackness; but is longsuffering to us-ward, not willing that any should perish, but that all should come to repentance." *(II Peter 3:9, KJV)*

It's amazing how 'Ecclesiastes 8:11-like' we can be, when only one generation away we see our parents experiencing the negative consequences of unhealthy living, or these 'sentences against an evil work.' How insane of us, as young people, to never conceive that we would ever be in the same shape as our parents, despite the fact we may be living in an even more unhealthy manner than they.

You may feel like you have lost 20, 30, 40, even 50 years of meaningful living, that your life up until now has been a waste. As harsh as it may sound, you may be exactly right. Your life may have been even worse than a waste. Maybe your life has had a negative impact on the world around you. But as I look back over the 30 years that I blew, I try to encourage myself in several ways.

One, the necessary sanctification and renewal process that God calls each of His followers to, at least for me, unfortunately, took 30 years. There may be a bit of a cop-out in that philosophy, but it seems to help me just the same.

Two, I try to encourage myself by being reminded that God can still accomplish great things with the rest of my life and in the lives of my family through me. There is plenty of good left for me to do and experience.

Third, I hope that God will somehow accomplish all that He desired in my life despite my lost time, that somehow He could use even the bad things of my past to contribute to the positive efforts of my present and future life; somehow 'restoring the years that the locust hast eaten.'

And fourth, God was very merciful to me in terms of the level of consequences my sinful life brought me. As bad as it was, it could have been much worse.

Is a lifetime of soda, milkshakes, and cookies worth all that regret? Is giving into a sinful lifestyle what God wants for you? Is that what you want for yourself? Did you want to live your life overweight? Living an overweight life is living a life where a death has occurred as we have submitted ourselves to the lusts of our flesh.

"... every man is tempted, when he is drawn away of his own lust, and enticed. Then when lust hath conceived, it bringeth forth sin; and sin, when it is finished, bringeth forth death. Do not err, my beloved brethren." (James 1:14-16, KJV)

Another reason we end up in such poor shape in life, whether physically and/or in other areas of life, is because we are more than willing to take advantage of God's patience and longsuffering towards us. That is, at least we are hopeful (wishful) that He will always be patient and longsuffering with us.

"The Lord is not slack concerning his promise, as some men count slackness; but is longsuffering to us-ward, not willing that any should perish, but that all should come to repentance." (II Peter 3:9, KJV)

Although this verse is speaking specifically about salvation it still gives a glimpse into the long-suffering character of God.

When I consider all of the abuse we heap upon our bodies I am shocked that we can even live 70 to 80 years. It doesn't even make scientific sense to me. But that doesn't mean that we will not suffer, and have not suffered, from the consequences of our sin. As we saw in Psalm 90:7-12, and as we are experiencing today, in addition to not living the full 120 years that God ultimately desires for each of us, we still will have to suffer through fatigue and degenerative disease. So God's longsuffering is not about giving us more time to disobey. God's longsuffering is about giving us every opportunity to turn back to Him.

I don't want to live my life as a moan, as a whimper (Psalm 90:7-12), because I am unwilling to submit my life to God's wisdom and leading. And I know you don't want that either.

In any event, despite popular opinion and practice within the Christian Community, God cares greatly about your physical health. The Bible is filled with passages addressing diet, rest, exercise, medical care, fasting, and cleanliness, as well as such indirect components of physical health as forgiveness, love, purposeful living, etc. I refer to these as components of the Biblical Doctrine of Physical Health.

When we walk in disobedience to these directives/commands of God, although the consequences do not occur overnight, Ecclesiastes

8:11 tells us that we will one day 'pay the piper' and reap what we have sown.

"Do not be deceived, God is not mocked; for whatever a man sows, that he will also reap. For he who sows to his flesh will of the flesh reap corruption, but he who sows to the Spirit will of the Spirit reap everlasting life. And let us not grow weary while doing good, for in due season we shall reap if we do not lose heart." (Galatians 6:7-9, KJV)

"... be sure your sin will find you out." (Numbers 32:23, KJV)

I have heard it said that sin will always take us where we didn't want to go, further than we agreed to go, and will cost us more than we wanted to pay.

The 'evil fruit of our evil ways' is nowhere more obviously displayed than in our poor physical health and reduced lifespan. The fact that we cannot hide this evil fruit is the very reason we are so resistant to acknowledge our 'secret sin' (Psalm 90:7-12).

"For a good tree does not bear bad fruit, nor does a bad tree bear good fruit. For every tree is known by its own fruit..." (Luke 6:43-44, NKJV, BibleGateway.com)

If we will acknowledge our sin of living in disobedience to God's Word regarding diet and health, our secret sin, and consider the years of others around is, relative to both quality and quantity, we will better equipped and motivated to avoid the consequences of that sin in our lives.

We have also found ourselves in this place because we have forgotten who we are as Believers. We have forgotten that Jesus came that we might live above our fleshly natures. We have failed to acknowledge that we are now heirs of God, intended to be set apart from the base things of this world in favor of the higher things of God. We have wallowed in the mud when God wants us to soar above all the nations.

Another reason why we have come to such a poor state, in health, body weight, and lifespan, is because we do not fully acknowledge just how filthy are our dietary practices are. Just take a few moments to consider the types of garbage, and how much garbage, the average American consumes, shoving down French fries, Debbie Cakes, and soda day in and day out.

I know we Americans tend to think of ourselves as very clean. It's those people in other countries that are not clean, right? But from a diet and health standpoint, we have given into filthy living. I don't care how many baths a person takes, how much perfume and lotion they apply to their body, and how fancy they might dress, a body that is 50, 75, 100+ pounds overweight is filthy, at least on the inside, and has followed filthy dietary practices to get there. I know that sounds harsh, but to abuse our bodies to the point of this type of excess reflects a filthiness in our souls and a resulting filthiness in our bodies. Consider these passages as you reflect on my comments.

"There is a generation that are pure in their own eyes, and yet is not washed from their filthiness." (Proverbs 30:12, KJV)

"Having therefore these promises, dearly beloved, let us cleanse ourselves from all filthiness of the flesh and spirit, perfecting holiness in the fear of God." (II Corinthians 7:1, KJV)

"Wherefore lay apart all filthiness and superfluity of naughtiness, and receive with meekness the engrafted word which is able to save your souls." (James 1:21, KJV)

Another strong word to go along with filthiness is perverseness. Our lack of dietary holiness, and even our unwillingness to admit that such a thing exists, is an absolute perversion. It is a perversion of Scripture and the very character of God that we have used to justify the destruction of our bodies through an unhealthy, unholy diet.

"… the perversion of transgressors shall destroy them." (Proverbs 11:3, KJV)

Let's add another word to describe our unhealthy, unholy diets; naughtiness. Relative to diet and health, the Church has behaved as a naughty, disobedient child.

"… transgressors shall be taken in their own naughtiness." (Proverbs 11:6, KJV)

Our unhealthy, unholy diets are also mischievous. Our pride keeps us in mischief as it spiritually enables us to argue against any reason or truth presented to us, and to live in denial of any truth that would 'dare' to require us to change our ways.

"… he that hardeneth his heart shall fall into mischief." (Proverbs 28:14, KJV)

An unhealthy, unholy diet is filthy, perverse, naughty, and mischievous. That is why the Church is tired, sick, overweight, and living only a fraction of the years God intended.

Here are a few final comments God might provide to answer the question, 'How did we get this way to start with?'

"The fear of the Lord is the beginning of knowledge: but fools despise wisdom and instruction." (Proverbs 1:7, KJV)

I think the 'fear of the Lord' involves a strong respect for Him. When we respect someone we tend to look to them for guidance. In effect, in the area of diet and health, the Church has failed to show God any respect whatsoever. We have been foolish in this regard. And because we have failed to respect God's wisdom and power concerning our diet and health, we have failed to depart from evil. We have failed to walk in dietary holiness and are now overweight and unhealthy.

"… by fear of the Lord men depart from evil." (Proverbs 16:6, KJV)

"He that diggeth a pit shall fall into it…" (Ecclesiastes 10:8, KJV)

"The fear of the Lord is the beginning of wisdom: a good understanding have all they that do his commandments…" (Psalm 111:10, KJV)

In this case we have dug the pit with our forks, literally. I love how God can state some things in the most common-sense way. And God might offer in conclusion…

"They would have none of my counsel: they despised all my reproof. Therefore shall they eat of the fruit of their own way, and be filled with their own devices. For the turning away of the simple shall slay them, and the prosperity of fools shall destroy them. But whoso hearkeneth unto me shall dwell safely, and shall be quiet from fear of evil." (Proverbs 1:30-33, KJV)

If we will hearken unto God's voice, and not turn away from His dietary directives, then we will have no need to fear the evil of an unhealthy and overweight body as caused by an unhealthy diet.

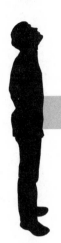
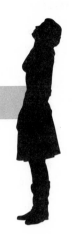

Chapter 13

The Physical – Emotional – Spiritual Connection

I think that God is especially concerned about your health and your body weight because of how the physical affects the spiritual. We talked earlier about how the spiritual (spiritual conditioning) ultimately affects the physical. But it is also important to understand that the physical affects the spiritual.

Your total being is made up of spirit, soul, and body, each component intricately interconnected with the other. Trying to separate the three components of your being as if one is not part of the other is one way in which the Christian Community has been able to live in denial with regard to the application of the Biblical Doctrine of Physical Health. This has been a foolish practice that has garnered serious consequences in our lives, physically, emotionally, and spiritually.

Your physical health and body weight will have a serious impact on your ability to serve God and others, and to walk righteously in every area of your life. This is certainly a good reason for God to be concerned with how you treat your body. And this is why God let you know that 'your body is not your own' (I Corinthians 6:19-20) and that He cares about what we eat (Leviticus 11 and Deuteronomy 14 – discussed later).

I think God knew that if we had free reign over our bodies we would work to destroy them, to include negatively impacting our spiritual life. For those who refuse to acknowledge that their bodies are not their own, and for those who believe the destruction of their bodies is some kind of freedom we have in Christ, God's concern has proved valid. If left to ourselves we have proven we will follow very unhealthy practices.

I would dare to guess that at least 50% of our spiritual potential is left untapped due to poor physical health and excess weight. This untapped potential comes in three forms; outward witness, service, and behavior.

Witness

As stated earlier, an unhealthy and overweight person is a poor witness to the world of the wisdom and power of God that is available to each of us, of the wisdom and power of God that we claim with our mouths. I realize this may sound like a harsh statement, but it is true nonetheless.

Walking around 50+ pounds overweight with a soda and candy bar in our hands communicates to the world that we lack self-control, that we lack a sense of purpose in our lives, that we lack energy/vitality, that we are lacking in the social graces, and that we are not very intelligent. Nobody will be beating down the Church doors to learn how to 'get some of that.'

God is very desirous that we reach the world for Christ. God desires that all be saved and that none should perish. Being a positive witness is an important part of reaching the world for Christ. This is why God calls us to be a peculiar people, a people who live their lives in such a way that the fruit of our living is beneficial to the Believer and attractive to the unbeliever.

"The Lord is... not willing that any should perish, but that all should come to repentance." (II Peter 3:9, KJV)

*"For thou art an holy people unto the L*ORD *thy God, and the L*ORD *hath chosen thee to be a peculiar people unto himself, above all the nations that are upon the earth."* (Deuteronomy 14:2, KJV)

I love the cry that Russell Crowe makes in the movie The Gladiator, 'What we do in life echoes in eternity!' I think there is some truth to be found in that statement, most especially as it applies to leading the world to Jesus Christ by our witness.

Service

You are also called to live a life of service, serving God and others. God knows that to effectively do that you need to be in good physical condition. No wonder God is so concerned about your diet and your health. It is an important tool for your kingdom work. God wants you to be furnished unto all good works. An unhealthy and overweight body is not furnished unto all good works.

"All scripture is given by inspiration of God, and is profitable for doctrine, for reproof, for correction, for instruction in righteousness: that the man of God may be perfect, thoroughly furnished unto all good works." (II Timothy 3:16, KJV)

God also tells us that your faith is of little practical value here on earth if there are no good works that follow. Your ability and potential to perform good works in your life will be negatively affected by poor health and excess weight. A life without good works is vain (a waste). Don't let your unwillingness to walk in Godly wisdom regarding diet and health stand between you and a meaningful (not vain) life.

"But wilt thou know, O vain man, that faith without works is dead?" (James 2:20, KJV)

Behavior

How you react to the world around you also impacts your spiritual potential. All things being the same, your body's hormonal and chemical balance, as directly affected by your physical health, will either enable you to respond calmly and positively to others or it will cause you to respond harshly and negatively to others.

Responding harshly and negatively to others is an act of sin that harms you spiritually, provides a poor example for other Believers, and inhibits your witness to others. And regardless of how determined you might be to respond in love and kindness to others, if your 'nerves are fried' due to an unhealthy lifestyle, you will have a hard time achieving that. God knows this. This is another reason why God is so concerned about what you eat and your physical health.

It's fairly easy to understand that an emotionally disturbed person will have a greater tendency to fall into sin than one who one who is not. This is true whether the person is emotionally disturbed because of poor thinking or the person is emotionally disturbed because of the hormonal/chemical issues that arise due to poor health. The pathway from wonderful to witch, from gentlemen to jerk, is often paved with soda, candy, cookies, fried foods, and caffeine.

I believe that the greatest majority of the cases of depression we are seeing in this country are simply the result of a poorly functioning body, primarily that of the endocrine and central nervous systems. I have heard it said that up to 70% of today's mental wards would empty out within a matter of months if the patients were simply taken off their diets of refined sugars, refined flours, caffeine, and medications.

It is also worth noting that your spiritual experience is not compartmentalized. What I mean by that is each area of your Christian walk affects every other area of your Christian walk. All areas of your Christian walk work together to form a whole spiritual experience.

What does this mean relative to achieving your ideal body weight? Your ability to walk in obedience to God's Word regarding diet, your spiritual conditioning, will either be positively or negatively impacted by the level of obedience to God with which you are walking in other areas of your life.

You can't expect success in applying the Biblical principles of diet and weight loss when you are disrespecting your spouse, not loving your children, viewing sexually explicit material on television or in print, stealing from your employer, not giving financially to God's work, etc. As I mentioned before, God is interested in the development of your whole person, your entire spiritual experience.

This is why I urged you at the beginning of the book to continue with regular Bible study and prayer in addition to any book study you might have embarked upon that only addresses one area of Scripture. This is what spiritual conditioning is all about, developing your overall spiritual strength and motivation (fruit of the Spirit) that you can apply to every area of your life. God wants all of you, not just your eating habits. But make no mistake. He clearly wants you to eat in obedience to His Word. What you eat does matter to God.

God wants you to understand your body is not your own, that He is the commander and chief of all things fitness in your life. God wants you to understand that you are made up of three interconnected components; spirit, soul, and body. God wants you to understand that the spirit affects the soul and body, and that the body affects the soul and spirit. God wants you to understand that your spiritual experience cannot be compartmentalized. And God wants you to know that what you eat, your health, and your body weight do matter to Him.

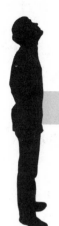
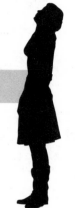

Chapter 14

God's Diet Plan – The Basic Outline

In Ecclesiastes 10:17 God has managed to communicate in 10 words most, if not all, of the instruction regarding diet that you will ever need. The rest is largely just common sense. You can literally exchange that entire room of dietary materials we spoke about earlier for only 10 words from God.

"… eat in due season, for strength, and not for drunkenness." (Ecclesiastes 10:17, KJV)

Ecclesiastes 10:17 is the best dietary summary in the world. In only 10 words God has been able to more powerfully, more succinctly, more accurately, and less convolutedly provide us with His dietary wisdom. We could put a host of the best dietary books ever written together and not reap more wisdom than God has provided us in these few words. I did promise you that the Bible is the greatest health and weight loss book ever written!

In these 10 words God tells us what you are to eat, when you are to eat, how much you are to eat, and why you are to eat. Ecclesiastes 10:17 alone, a single verse, hits on all four of these topics. Let's unpack these 10 words.

Eat in Due Season
You should eat when your body is calling for food (when you are hungry).

It doesn't matter if you are 100+ pounds overweight. If you are trying to fight off hunger pangs in an effort to lose weight then stop resisting right now and go get something to eat (something healthy).

This is how you work with your body and the intelligence with which God designed it. Trust the messages your body sends you. Over time, as your body gets the nutrients it's craving, and as your body balances itself chemically and hormonally, hunger will occur less and less frequently and the amount of food required to satisfy your hunger will decrease as well.

On the flip-side, maybe you are not dieting at all (you shouldn't 'diet' to begin with), but rather, you are in your 'normal eating mode,' which is eating when you are not hungry at all. You are eating just because you are bored or someone has placed a plate of something in front of you. This is not the time to eat. This is not eating in 'due season.'

This portion of the verse addresses 'when you are to eat.' It also addresses emotional eating / 'why you are to eat' in that the purpose for eating is not to quench our negative emotions (sadness or boredom), but to nourish our bodies when the time comes, in due season. We are to turn to God with our emotional struggles, not food.

Eat For Strength

We are to eat in order to nourish and strengthen our bodies. Junk non-foods like soda, pastries, candy, and the like do not nourish or 'strengthen' our bodies. These things poison, destroy, and 'weaken' our bodies. Obedience to this portion of the verse alone would have an enormous effect on the incidence of various degenerative diseases that are at epidemic and 'plague' proportions in our society today. These three words alone, 'eat for strength,' are enough to take you to your ideal body weight.

It is important to note that the definition of food is <u>not</u> any substance that can be consumed, tastes good, and doesn't kill you in less than 24 hours. We call the unhealthy stuff 'junk food', but it is not food at all. By God's definition and creative evidence, if it doesn't nourish and strengthen your body, then it is not food.

God's foods are those substances created, designed, and prescribed by God to nourish your body. If a substance does not nourish your body, then it is not food. Refined sugars, refined flours, and hydrogenated oils, for example, not only do not nourish your body, but actually work to destroy it. Food, or God's food, since there is no other, is always nourishing to your body.

What we call junk food is nothing more than chemical derivatives of things that once might have been food, but are now poisons. This is much like the fact that heroin is a chemical derivative of morphine, morphine is a chemical derivative of opium, and opium is a chemical derivative of the poppy seed (God's original creation). Man can take God's creation and convert it into something as destructive to mankind as heroin. This perversion of God's creation is the same evil that occurs when man takes God's creation (sugar cane, beets, corn) and converts it into refined sugars. Both heroin and refined sugars are toxic poisons to the body.

If you were given a pile of burnt flower ashes and told to decorate your home with it, you would not be accommodating. The ashes were once flowers, but because of the 'process' to which they were subjected, they no longer maintain the properties of flowers to beautify and serve your home. You would not consider the ashes to be flowers. Yet that is exactly how we treat the substances we eat. The only screening criteria is often how it tastes, not whether or not it has the properties of food to nourish our bodies.

Please get this. There is no such thing as junk food or unhealthy food. Either it is food or it is some chemical garbage that man has made to taste good. God defines what is food and what is not food, not man. This is true just as God determines what is (man-woman) and what is not (man-man and woman-woman) marriage. What God has provided and calls food are those things that nourish our bodies, not those man-created things that poison our bodies.

I have been asked, 'What is the difference between eating the sugar cane and eating the refined sugar created from it?' Here is my answer to that question.

Sugarcane – God's designed and prescribed food
Refined sugar – Chemical derivative of God's designed and prescribed food

Sugarcane – non-addictive
Refined sugar – addictive

Sugarcane – contains fiber to control blood sugar levels
Refined sugar – contains no fiber to control blood sugar levels, which leads to a variety of strains on the body that damage our pancreas, adrenals, liver, etc., forming the basis for degenerative health

Sugarcane – contains nutrients to serve the body and to help the body process its carbohydrates into energy
Refined sugar – contains practically no nutrients to serve the body and literally must steal nutrients from the body in order to process its carbohydrates into energy, which leads to degenerative health

Sugarcane – nourishes the body
Refined sugar – poisons the body

The properties of the sugarcane to serve your body, as God designed it to do for you, no longer exist in the perverted form of refined sugar, which damages your body. Refined sugars are not food. And they are more than 'empty calories.' Refined sugars are 'negative calories,' literally stealing nutrients from the body.

The refinement process strips the fiber and nutrients from the food. This is desirable from the manufacturer's standpoint for several reasons.

One, various nutrients and oils in God's foods often do not lend to giving the food a long shelf-life. In order for the manufacturer to reduce costs and increase profits, they turn to increasing shelf-life. The shelf-life of a food is increased by removing many of the nutrients and oils via processing/refinement.

Two, by removing the fiber from the food, a more concentrated 'flavor' can be created. And three, relative to removing the fiber, more applications are created. For example, by removing the fiber from corn, the manufacturer can create a substance (high fructose corn syrup, for example) that can be more easily added to other processed foods. Or in the case of something like simple refined, granulated sugar, the consumer can easily scoop out spoonfuls of the stuff for its addition to coffee, cakes, cookies, and the like.

By the way, the extraction process is more than just taking away nutrients, which is bad enough all by itself. The manufacturers will also add various chemicals and gases to the food in order to expedite or more deeply refine the food. Although they may argue that these chemicals and gases are removed further down the line in the refinement process, traces of these chemicals and gases remain. So not only is this processed chemical incompatible and poisonous to your body, but additional poisons are actually added as well. So the refinement process involves turning God's foods into poison and adding more poisons on top of that.

Through refinement man can concentrate the intensity of God's flavorings beyond what He intended. For example, man can concentrate the amount of natural sugars God added to a pound of His food down to a fraction of an ounce of refined sugar. This contributes to the addictive power of the substance.

I believe God knew that to go beyond a certain point of 'taste' would only lead to greater tendencies toward addictive eating. But even as I say that, I must mention that when you get yourself off perverted non-foods, the foods of God begin to taste so much better. For me, an orange and an apple are deliciously and incredibly sweet. There is no candy or ice-cream that would taste any better. As a matter of fact, once you have cleansed your palate with a few weeks of God's foods, candy and ice-cream have an unpleasing taste about them. But if you were to forge ahead and eat them a few times over a period of a week or so, you would find yourself enjoying them just like you once did. Good tends to begat good. Bad tends to begat bad.

But isn't that principle always true? Isn't that a spiritual principle? When we focus on the things of Satan, the things of God always seem to lose their 'flavor' in comparison. When we turn away from the things of Satan towards the things of God, we find that life and His ways become 'sweeter' by the day.

So why are refined sugars produced and consumed? They are produced because of the greed and lust of mankind. It is just that simple. And Satan wants to destroy you with this greed and lust.

"The thief cometh not, but for to steal, and to kill, and to destroy..." (John 10:10, KJV)

This portion of Ecclesiastes 10:17 speaks to 'what we are to eat' and 'why we are to eat.'

Not for Drunkenness

We are not to allow the poor quality of our diet, or the excess quantity of our diet, to leave us groggy mentally and physically. God wants us to feel good, to be alert, and to be productive. 'Drunken' eating, which may be from unhealthy dietary choices and/or overeating, is against God's will for your life. This portion of the verse addresses 'how much you are to eat,' 'what you are to eat,' and 'why you are to eat.'

Ecclesiastes 10:17 cuts through all of the non-sense and ever-changing philosophies of the weight loss industry. It eliminates the burden of counting calories and fat grams. These complicated and self-focused ways are clearly not of God, having been orchestrated by Satan through man's foolishness and self-reliance.

In the introduction section of *The Gabriel Method*, Jon Gabriel does a great job of expressing the sentiments of Ecclesiastes 10:17, although he doesn't give any direct reference to God or the Bible concerning the technical wisdom he had obtained through study and personal experimentation.

I strongly recommend you read his book at some point. Jon lost 225 pounds in a manner and with the wisdom that resonates with all things God, again, although he didn't attribute that wisdom to seeking God directly.

Excerpts from *The Gabriel Method* that work well to explain and exemplify the message of Ecclesiastes 10:17 include...

Eat in Due Season – "I stopped treating every hunger pang as a battle. If I was hungry, I would eat, and if I wasn't hungry, I wouldn't eat." (*The Gabriel Method*, xvi, Jon Gabriel)

Eat for Strength – "So, in actuality, one of the reasons I was hungry all the time was that I was starving for nutrients. I was starving my body. Since it couldn't use the food I was eating, it just stayed hungry and continued to starve." (*The Gabriel Method*, xvi, Jon Gabriel)

Not for Drunkenness – "And it wasn't just my body that was starving. I was starving in every aspect of my life. I was starving mentally, emotionally, and spiritually. I was not listening to or following my heart. I was living according to a preconceived notion of what my life was supposed to be. My heart was telling me to go in a different direction altogether, and I wasn't listening." (*The Gabriel Method*, xvii, Jon Gabriel)

God's Word is amazing. It is relevant, timeless, and cuts straight to the core of any issue. It's all in there if you want to find it.

"... he that hath ears to hear, let him hear." (Luke 8:8, KJV)

Jesus is asking you to challenge yourself with the question, 'can I handle the truth?' This is a vital point of self-introspection (getting real with yourself before God), one the Church urgently needs to perform in the area of the Biblical Doctrine of Physical Health.

Are you not impressed with God's ability to express so much wisdom in only 10 words? Are you disregarding the dietary instruction God provided for you here in favor of a mountain of diet books and schemes written and developed by man? Are you still hoping to find a magic pill that will not require you to control your diet in accordance with Ecclesiastes 10:17? I trust that by now your answer to each of these questions is 'no.'

God's ways are always simple, effective, never-changing, and freeing, although challenging at times. Satan's ways are always complicated, ineffective, ever-changing, and enslaving. If that doesn't describe the wisdom of man, and its results, found in the fitness world today then I don't know what does.

"For God is not the author of confusion, but of peace..." (I Corinthians 14:33, KJV)

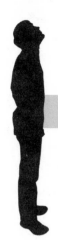
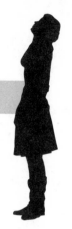

Chapter 15

The Sober Life

The Bible is so saturated with passages that address gluttony and drunkenness (in food and/or drink) that I will let God's Word do more talking in this chapter than I have in any other. It seemed beneficial to just let these passages flow. Carefully and prayerfully meditate upon the Scripture references in this chapter as you consider dietary holiness and your journey to your ideal body weight.

The Bible calls us to 'be sober'. It is interesting that God equates an unhealthy diet with drunkenness. For example, many children and youth today are either hyped-up on refined sugars and caffeine (drunk) or limp, non-responsive noodles with poor attitudes, fatigue, and a lack of motivation (hung-over).

Even apart from large quantities of food, we can also get drunk on moderate quantities of junk non-foods. Who hasn't experienced a temporary high from downing some soda and cake only to be hit with a crash soon after? It doesn't take much of the bad stuff.

In our modern world, we are living anything but the sober life. The sober life is not an obsessed, addicted, frenzied, self-focused, disoriented life, which is exactly how many of us live. That is a drunken life. Is it any wonder why we have trouble controlling our diets?

We are often not living a sober life. In this country we are getting 'smashed' every day on not just food and alcohol, but also on music, television, holiday rituals, sexual stimulation, entertainment, technology, parties, achievements, athletics, and making money. Getting away from our tendency towards drunkenness requires a total life makeover, not just a change in our diets.

"… that we may lead a quiet and peaceable life in all godliness and honesty." (*I Timothy 2:2, KJV*)

"… return ye now every man from his evil way, and amend your doings, and go not after other gods…" (*Jeremiah 35:15, KJV*)

"But take heed to yourselves, lest your hearts be weighed down with carousing, drunkenness, and cares of this life…" (*Luke 21:34, KJV*)

"Teaching us that, denying ungodliness and worldly lusts, we should live soberly, righteously, and godly, in this present world." (*Titus 2:12, KJV*)

There is not enough food in the world, or a stomach capacity large enough, to satisfy the spirit of gluttony. The physical limitations of our stomachs will not allow dietary drunkenness to keep us 'totaled' as often as the glutton might desire. The spirit of gluttony is an unquenchable fire. When we can't escape any further with food, we will find another addiction to act as back-up. It's a form of Maslow's Hierachy of Needs. The tendency of the glutton is to keep working down the list.

"When I had fed them to the full, then they committed adultery." (*Jeremiah 5:7, KJV*)

"The righteous eateth to the satisfying of his soul: but the belly of the wicked shall want." (*Proverbs 13:25, KJV*)

"Their sorrows shall be multiplied that hasten after another god…" (*Psalm 16:4, KJV*)

And when we find ourselves unable to get to another addictive behavior quick enough because of circumstances we find that we become quite depressed and irritable. We are irritated by the inability to medicate against the pain of running from God and living a purposeless life in those times.

I recall a cartoon that involved a dog-catcher, a dog, a cat, two mice, and a warehouse full of cheese. It began with the two mice, each completely obsessed with eating cheese. The two mice stumbled upon a warehouse full of cheese. They ate and ate until both their stomachs looked like watermelons. Being so full, the mice realized that they no longer had the desire/ability to eat any more cheese, which had been their sole pleasure in life previously. So the mice decided that life wasn't worth living anymore.

These mice walked up to a cat and asked the cat to eat them. The cat, whose sole pleasure in life was to chase mice, realized that his desire/ability to chase mice had been taken away. So he decided that life wasn't worth living anymore. The cat then walked up to a dog and asked the dog to eat him. The dog, whose sole pleasure in life was chasing cats, realized that his desire/ability to chase cats had been taken away. So the dog decided life wasn't worth living. In the final scene of the cartoon the dog is chasing after a dog-catcher's truck, the cat is chasing after the dog, and the two mice are chasing after the cat.

The emotional pains we are feeling have to be dealt with and/or drowned out one way or the other. If we try to count on some pleasure, or pleasures, we will often find ourselves feeling like life isn't worth living anytime we aren't suckling on that pacifier of addictive behavior.

We have to decide if we are going to turn to the Spirit of God and the pursuit of purpose that can satisfy, or keep turning to the spirit of gluttony and the pursuit of pleasure that can never satisfy.

"... chose you this day whom ye will serve..." (Joshua 24:15, KJV)

We typically think of Sodom and Gomorrah as being synonymous with sexual perversion, which it was, but look again and see their gluttony for food. Pride (a lack of humility before God / not understanding your body is not your own) can lead to gluttony, and then gluttony will lead to fatigue/idleness.

"Look, this was the iniquity of your sister Sodom: She and her daughter had pride, fullness of food, and abundance of idleness..." (Ezekiel 16:49, KJV)

Gluttony destroys the health of the body because your body is not equipped to handle an overload of food. An overload of food creates a huge energy drain on the body, as your digestive system seeks out every available energy reserve in its effort to deal with the huge challenge. This creates what God calls a state of drunkenness, or grogginess and lethargy as we might say, as the energies required by your brain and basic motor systems are stolen away to deal with the processing of the excess food.

We know today that law enforcement is cracking down on drunk driving. I believe drunkenness while driving may be the leading cause of violent deaths in this country. You may not have ever thought about gluttony producing a state of drunkenness in the body and mind as well.

Studies have been conducted that correlate certain levels of fatigue and poor health to the condition of legal intoxication. The point of such studies is to demonstrate that the extended response time of someone who is tired and/or in some other state of poor health can be equal to that of someone at a legal level of alcohol intoxication.

We can all relate to that reality. Who has not eaten too much for lunch and found themselves left moving slowly and sluggishly, both physically and mentally? Coffee makers don't have a problem with our mid-day gluttony (drunkenness). I would suspect that the consumption of caffeinated beverages an hour or so after such meals contributes to a large percentage of their sales.

The biggest desire in America seems to be weight-loss. What

an emotional nightmare for us, that we would be so gluttonous and overweight, worshipping food, yet live in a world, to include the Church, that equally worships the body-beautiful. But such is the life of those given to living apart from God's commands.

"... the way of the transgressor is hard." (Proverbs 13:15, KJV)

We often joke about how much we may have eaten recently or how stuffed we might be. I have heard it said that what we laugh at today, we accept tomorrow. God's people have long since determined the gluttonous lifestyle to be acceptable. And we are foolish to have done so.

"Fools make a mock at sin..." (Proverbs 14:9, KJV)

The Church is so far gone in the area of dietary deception that jokes about how we eat are made all the time. We joke about eating too much. We joke about all the garbage we ate. Although we would prefer not to be overweight, we even joke about that. Just imagine if members of the Church walked around joking about the adulterous relationships they were in, the money they stole from others, the weekend of gossip they just enjoyed, or how drunk they got Friday night. Puts a whole new light on it, doesn't it?

The spirit of gluttony exists because deep-down we believe the lie that the more we can consume, the happier we will be, or at least the more pain we can bury. But the opposite is true. Fundamentally, the spirit of gluttony is similar to the spirit of greed. The soul of the glutton always wants more, yet is one that is left unsatisfied, unfulfilled, and impoverished; spiritually, emotionally, physically, and often financially.

"For the drunkard and glutton shall come to poverty..." (Proverbs 23:21, KJV)

"He that loveth silver will not be satisfied with silver, nor he that loveth abundance with increase..." (Ecclesiastes 5:10, KJV)

"So are the ways of everyone that is greedy of gain, which taketh away the life of the owners thereof." (Proverbs 1:19, KJV)

We must run to God with our emotional struggles, not food. We are to worship Him and no other god. And we must accept that difficult times are part of life, not something from which to seek out every conceivable way from which to escape. Consider the following Scriptures in order to gain a Godly perspective on your struggles and what God expects from us.

"Thou shalt worship no other gods before me." (Hosea 13:4, KJV)

"Humble yourselves therefore under the mighty hand of God, that He may exalt you in due time: casting all your care upon Him; for He careth for you. Be sober... knowing that the same afflictions are accomplished in your brethren that are in the world." (I Peter 5:6-9, KJV)

"... in the world ye shall have tribulation, but be of good cheer. I have overcome the world." (John 16:33, KJV)

"My brethren, count it all joy when ye fall into various trials; knowing this, that the trying of your faith worketh patience. But let patience have her perfect work, that ye may be perfect and entire, wanting nothing." (James 1:2-4, KJV)

Difficulties in life are guaranteed. How you decide you want to handle them is up to you. Will you turn to God or will you continue to turn to food and junk non-foods. Will you choose the bounty of a purposeful life filled with God's best for you, or will you choose to scrape by on the mere crumbs of an addicted, pleasure-focused life, often feeling like those mice that had just as soon let the cat eat them?

I know that you can overcome gluttony in your life, and not only in the area of diet. You can live a sober life. You can have control over your diet instead of your diet having control over you. God has provided everything you need to live in victory.

Focus on the fact that your body is not your own. Seek God's wisdom concerning diet. Strengthen yourself through spiritual conditioning. And start choosing purpose over pleasure. In no time flat the hold of unhealthy eating on your life will exist no more, and your journey to your ideal body weight will be well on its way.

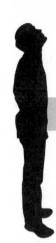
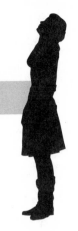

Chapter 16

God's Diet Plan – Digging Deeper

In the chapter 'A Righteous Motivation is Needed to Reach Your Ideal Body Weight' we discussed Deuteronomy 14:2. In this verse we learned that God's people are called to live by God's commandments, to be a holy people. And we learned that the positive results of obedience to God's commandments would be so impressive, standing out 'above all the nations,' that we would be blessed and the world would be drawn to God in the process.

Let's now add Deuteronomy 14:3 and consider the directive that God gave us in order to achieve these 'positive results' in our lives.

"For thou art an holy people unto the Lord *thy God, and the* Lord *hath chosen thee to be a peculiar people unto himself, above all the nations that are upon the earth. Thou shalt not eat any abominable thing." (Deuteronomy 14:2-3, KJV)*

The very next verse after God has called us to live a life that gets the attention of the rest of the world, He then addresses diet. This is huge!!! God is telling us that obedience to His diet plan (dietary holiness) is a critical component of making the Church stand out above all the nations that are upon the Earth as a testimony to God's wisdom and power. And is this passage not an incredible testimony to the fact that God cares greatly about what you eat? Your diet is no small matter to God.

This is how we can glorify God (draw the attention of others to Him). We already saw from I Corinthians 6:19-20 that God commands us to 'glorify Him in our bodies.'

Fitness experts are always contending that their fitness plan will give you positive results. God's fitness plan promises to give His people positive results that will make us stand out to the rest of the world. Those are staggering results! Don't miss this. This is mind-boggling. This is what the Church has available to it if we will obey God's commands, specifically, eating what God says we are to eat and not eating what God says we are not to eat.

Talk about a testimony to the truth that what we eat matters to God. Our dietary practices can be the very difference between God's people standing out, being a positive example to the world, and His people acting like the prodigal son, wallowing in the mud with everyone else. Is the Church willing to turn back to God with regard to diet in order to experience this type of impact in its life and in the lives of those watching us, the world? Are you willing to turn back to God with regard to diet in order to experience this type of impact in your life and in the lives of those looking to you for answers to life's questions?

Imagine a Church that is healthier than any other demographic on the planet, each member living at their ideal body weight, and living significantly longer than any other demographic on the planet. You want to talk about a powerful evangelical tool! The world would be beating down the doors to our churches trying to find out what we were doing differently, why we were doing it differently, and Who told us to do it differently; reaching more people for Christ in this modern era than ever before in history! That is what is at stake here.

God goes on to tell us which animal meats are okay for us to eat and which animal meats are not okay (an abomination/offense to God). For example, in Deuteronomy 14, God goes on to tell us that we should not eat pork. A similar type of listing of clean (okay) and unclean (not okay) animal meats are found in Leviticus 11.

We can see in Deuteronomy 14:2 that this discussion of diet constitutes a condition for holy living (a holy people). Now take a look at Leviticus 11:44.

"For I am the Lord your God: ye shall therefore sanctify yourselves, and ye shall be holy, for I am holy: neither shall ye defile yourselves with any manner of creeping thing that creepeth upon the earth." (Leviticus 11:44, KJV)

Sanctify means that God's people are to be 'set apart'. We discussed earlier that the word 'peculiar' in Deuteronomy 14:2 doesn't mean God's people are to be doing strange things without purpose only to get the world's attention. Similarly, God is not calling His people to be 'set apart' in that they should do strange things without purpose for the sole goal of differentiating His people from the rest of the world in that way. The point is that through obedience to God's dietary directives His people will be 'set apart' from the rest of the World with respect to appearance, body weight, health, and lifespan.

We also see another reference to God's dietary directives as a condition for holy living. We can see that God does not want us to defile (harm) our bodies with unclean, toxic, unhealthy things. To not defile ourselves means that we are not to put anything in our bodies that would be unhealthy for it. To defile your body is to make it unhealthy.

Most in the Church today contend that this list of approved and unapproved animal meats no longer applies to us, but only to God's people during that time period. This is dietary deception at work. I will make several comments to the contrary...

1) An understanding of the terms clean and unclean regarding animal meats was understood all the way back in Genesis 7:2 when God instructed Noah as to how many of each to gather into the ark.

2) The issue of clean and unclean in this regard is purely a physical

issue/concern of God, medical if you will. With the exception of obedience to His directives concerning diet, there is no spiritual difference between a cow and a pig. However, there is a huge difference in the physical impact each will have on our bodies if consumed.

God calls a cow clean because of what it eats and how it digests its food, the result being a more pure musculature that is healthy for us to eat. God calls a pig unclean because of what it eats and how it digests its food, the result being a very impure, toxic musculature that is unhealthy for us to eat. Nothing more. Nothing less.

3) For those who want to contend that our freedoms in Christ somehow give us license to destroy our bodies with unhealthy diets that include pork and other unhealthy animal meats, I would ask, 'Why would God have cared about our physical health before Christ came and not give a rip about our physical health after Christ came?' That is utterly ridiculous. Consider II Corinthians 5:15.

"And that he died for all, that they which live should not henceforth live unto themselves, but unto him which died for them, and rose again." (II Corinthians 5:15, KJV)

Destroying your body via an unhealthy diet is living unto yourself, not unto God. And destroying your body is a right you forfeited when you accepted Jesus Christ as your Savior. You are now called to be a good steward of your body, just as you are called to be a good steward of your family, finances, and time.

4) There is nothing that Jesus Christ accomplished on the cross that made pork, for example, any less unhealthy than it was before the cross.

5) God addresses His dietary directives, in both Leviticus 11:44 and Deuteronomy 14:3, as a requirement for holy living. These were directives based on what was required to bless His people's physical bodies. There is nothing that changed regarding our physical bodies between then and now, nor God's concern for them.

I will address misinterpreted Scriptures used to contradict these points, but for now, suffice it to say that the motivation behind discounting these points is an adherence to the things of the flesh (death) and not the things of the Spirit (life).

I will leave it to you to study Leviticus 11 and Deuteronomy 14, but just know that these dietary directives of God still apply to you today. But what is the basic, all-encompassing principle that God is making in these passages? It is that He has clearly communicated that He is concerned about what we eat.

Does God's concern only apply to animal meats? As long as you avoid pork, catfish, and lobster, for example, can you eat all the refined sugars, refined flours, and hydrogenated oils you want? No. The specific point that God is making in these passages is that eating unhealthy things is an abomination/offense to Him. It goes way beyond the application to animal meats.

Remember, during this time in history, donuts and sodas did not exist. We have to understand the spirit of the principle 'God doesn't want us to put anything unhealthy in our bodies' to see that the consumption of refined sugars, refined flours, and hydrogenated oils is also an abomination/offense to God. This principle also applies to tobacco and illegal drugs, labeling them as sinful as well.

A quick aside... The refinement (perversion) processes than man eventually devised did not exist during Jesus' time. Over the centuries man devised more and more ways to accrue wealth, getting wealthier and wealthier through the years. Man's motivation to develop these money-making refinement processes was based on fleshly lust and greed. The nightmare of the history of man's perversion of God's foods through refining processes is no better communicated than by William Dufty in his book, *Sugar Blues*. Everyone needs to read his book. You will never be the same again after reading it.

Although there is nothing wrong with wealth in and of itself (if achieved righteously), it does offer the potential for uncontrolled, sinful behavior. I think we can see that played out very vividly in the area of unhealthy eating. The difference between successful living and unsuccessful living within the context of wealth comes down to being wise and being a fool.

The wise man can live successfully (eat healthy) within a wealthy environment. But the foolish man cannot. His very own wealth, or a wealthy environment, will only work to destroy him. And in case you are not aware, in this country, we all live in a wealthy environment. So be wise and not foolish.

"… the prosperity of fools shall destroy them." (Proverbs 1:32, KJV)

"A prudent man foreseeth the evil, and hideth himself; but the simple pass on, and are punished." (Proverbs 27:12, KJV)

Man oh man! Wisdom is screaming in the streets for someone to hear. Will you have ears to hear? Will you recognize evil by its evil fruit?

Why is eating unhealthy things an abomination/offense to God? It is because God cares for you and wants the best for you. And it is because God knows that eating unhealthy things will only work to harm you, and will produce results in your life (excess weight, for example) that do not glorify Him and His ways in front of the world.

God's angle here, for lack of a better term, is no different than it is with His directives regarding honesty, good work-ethic, giving, forgiveness, etc. God's Word is all about blessing you individually and reaching the world in the process. This is a consistent and central message throughout the Bible, applicable to every area of your life.

To contend that you are free to destroy your body with junk non-foods and gluttony because Christ's death freed you to do so is Biblical heresy, a complete contradiction to the character and ways of God presented throughout Scripture. If your body were a lawnmower, would the Master Mechanic want you to put engine-damaging substances in the gas tank?

The Biblical principle of Leviticus 11 and Deuteronomy 14 does not only apply to animal meats. The over-arching Biblical principle here is that God does not want you to place anything harmful in your body. So that extends the list from unclean animal meats to include refined flours, refined sugars, hydrogenated oils, and other toxic chemical products available for consumption in our modern world that work to destroy your health and keep you from your ideal body weight. And let's not forget that our bodies are not our own, to destroy as we might chose (I Corinthians 6:19-20).

What does abominable mean anyway? It sounds like one of those super-churchy words that no one really knows how to apply to practical living, or even thinks applies at all to us anymore for that matter. In a nutshell, 'abominable,' in laymen's terms, means nothing more than 'it is unhealthy for you and God doesn't want that for your life.' This is true whether that something is spiritually unhealthy, psychologically unhealthy, emotionally unhealthy, relationally unhealthy, physically unhealthy, or all of the above. To further clarify, consider Proverbs 6:16-19 as an example of additional things that God refers to as abominations.

"These six things doth the Lord hate: yea, seven are an abomination unto him: A proud look, a lying tongue, and hands that shed innocent blood, An heart that deviseth wicked imaginations, feet that be swift in running to mischief, A false witness that speaketh lies, and he that soweth discord among the brethren." (Proverbs 6:16-19, KJV)

God doesn't want you to eat a donut on Sunday morning any more than he wants you to greet the pastor with profanity. What we eat does matter to God.

"Whether therefore ye eat, or drink, or whatsoever ye do, do all to the glory of God." (I Corinthians 10:31, KJV)

"For I know the plans I have for you, declares the LORD, *plans to prosper you and not to harm you, plans to give you hope and a future." (Jeremiah 29:11, NIV, BibleGateway.com)*

Eating unhealthy things will make you overweight, keeping you from your ideal body weight. Being overweight does not glorify God. It does not draw positive attention to God. And glorifying Himself (drawing attention to Him and His ways) is something God desperately wants as He seeks to reach the world through your witness, blessing you with His best in the process. God wants you to reach and maintain your ideal body weight.

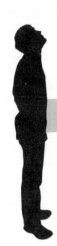
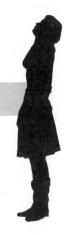

Chapter 17

The Biblical History & Changes in God's Diet Plan

The foods/diet that God prescribed for man changed two times, once when sin entered the world through Adam, and then later, when sin accrued to massive levels during the time of Noah.

The foods that God prescribed for man initially, in a sin-free world, were simply fruits and nuts/seeds. The original diet was very much a foraging diet.

"I have given you every herb bearing <u>seed</u>, which is upon the face of all the earth, and every tree, in which is the <u>fruit</u> of a tree yielding seed; to you it shall be meat." (Genesis 1:29, KJV)

So God gave man 'fruit' and 'seed' to eat. In Genesis 1:30, God goes on to say that in a sin-free world it was only the animals and insects that would eat the green herb, not man.

"And to every beast of the earth, and to every fowl of the air, and to every thing that creepeth upon the earth, wherein there is life, I have given every <u>green herb</u> for meat; and it was so." (Genesis 1:30, KJV)

So what happened to cause God to edit His diet plan? Sin happened. The entry of sin into this world had a degenerative effect on our bodies and/or on our environment. The nutrients found in the 'green herb' are needed now, to help us maintain good health under the new environmental conditions that sin has brought.

God also seems to communicate that 'bread' and 'cooking' would be part of the diet now as well. So don't let anybody try to convince you that you should avoid whole-grain breads.

"… thou shalt eat the <u>herb of the field</u>. In the sweat of thy face shalt thou eat <u>bread</u>…" (Genesis 3:18-19, KJV)

God did not intend for man to eat the herbs of the field. Also, God did not intend for man's diet to require cooking. It was man's sin that led to the necessity for this 'bitter blessing' of the herbs of the field and the 'work' of making bread.

I believe it helps people to know that they shouldn't be surprised that they want to avoid vegetables. When your child tells you they don't like vegetables, remind them, 'I know. You are not supposed to like green leafy vegetables. But these vegetables are a required bitter-blessing from God because of man's fall into sin, necessitating the need for the types of nutrients that only these vegetables can provide.' I believe God wants to work through our diets in this way to be a constant, daily reminder of the damage that sin can cause.

There is a huge life-lesson waiting for your children right there, for you and me as well. Through diet, whether relative to eating our vegetables or controlling the amount of food we eat, we have a daily opportunity to choose either the ways of God or the ways of man. I can't help but believe that diet is something that goes far beyond nourishment and enjoyment in God's plan for us.

God desires to use diet as a daily opportunity to draw His people closer to Him, and as a means whereby the Church can reach the world. A bit of careful thought in this regard quickly reveals that there is nothing else quite like the dietary process in our lives.

It is worth noting that the very fall of mankind into sin included a lust for food, a decision to eat something of which God did not approve. Your diet is no small matter. What you eat does matter to God.

But in any event, as you can see, it is God's will for your life (His dietary directive) that you eat green leafy vegetables (green herbs / herbs of the field). Here's yet another piece of your life that God has made His will for you evident.

It is important for your weight loss journey that you learn to be faithful in the little that you do know before you can expect for God to awaken you fully to His endless wisdom, whether with respect to a particular subject like diet, or the very purpose for which He placed you on this planet. It is important for your life overall to understand that. And this truth will prove important for your efforts to reach your ideal body weight.

I think that is how learning of God's 'total, more hidden will' for our lives, for lack of a better term, comes about or unfolds. It occurs as we are faithful to walk in the elements of His will for our lives of which we already know. Why would God want to reveal more for us 'not to do' anyway? So eat your green leafy vegetables, whether in the form of salad or cooked greens like spinach and collard greens.

While we are looking at the dietary changes that occurred due to our sinfulness, let's look at the final dietary change that God prescribed; animal meats. Up until the time of Noah humans did not eat animal meats, at least not by God's instruction. There had not even been any animal sacrifices, again, at least not by God's instruction. I suppose there could have been heathen peoples who killed, sacrificed, and ate animals before this time. I will leave that up to you to search that out if you so desire.

But with the environmental changes that took place as a result of the creation of the world flood, God determined it necessary to make another dietary change. And that change was for mankind to begin eating animals.

This mandate to begin eating animals wasn't because the Earth would have lacked enough vegetation to survive on when Noah's family initially left the ark, although that might have been true. If God had led them to store enough food to survive on for one year then He could have led them to store enough extra food to survive on for the number of months it might have taken for Noah and his family to find or plant and harvest some food subsequent to the flood. Also, God could have instructed man to eat animals for only a specific time, while the Earth's vegetation got up to speed. But we see no such direction.

Again, the environmental changes that would have occurred through the creation of the world flood that we discussed earlier (changes in oxygen levels, electromagnetic field, barometric presses, radiation, etc.) had a degenerative effect or impact on our bodies. These environmental changes put added strain on our bodies, enough to reduce the lifespan of man from 900+ down to 120.

In whatever form that strain came, God determined that the nutrients found in animal meat were necessary for our well-being (including red meat by the way). Science (good science) supports that there are certain nutrients that can only be found in animal meat, evidently nutrients not needed prior to the environmental conditions that developed post-flood. By the way, all good science ultimately works to support the wisdom of God found in the Bible.

Just imagine what it must have been like for those first people to learn to kill, cook, and eat animals. We take it for granted today, but that must have been a traumatic experience, both the killing and the eating. But then most of us don't really do that completely anyway. We are fairly far removed from at least the killing part of that equation, unless you are a hunter.

If we stop and think about it too much we could easily talk ourselves out of eating animals at all, largely out of our care and love for animals. And many people have done just that (vegetarians). Some of these vegetarians have even made it a life mission to convince others that killing animals for food is actually wrong and immoral, even evil. And I get that. I love animals too. If it were totally up to me to kill whatever animal meat my family ate we would probably never have anything but eggs.

But as heartfelt as their plea might be, unfortunately, this is man's wisdom, not God's. And just to be as open and honest as possible (God doesn't need me to protect Him anyway), the reality is that some of God's ways, at least in our human judgment, seem so harsh. But it is not ours to judge and determine appropriate life policy. That is God's business. It is our business to obey.

In short, the vegetarian life-style, as well-meaning as it might be, is not of God. And for those who simply believe that the vegetarian life-style is the healthiest life-style possible from a scientific standpoint, the God of all creation begs to differ.

Be sure to look to Leviticus 11 and Deuteronomy 14 for a list of animals that are clean to eat (part of God's diet plan) and which ones are unclean to eat (not part of God's diet plan). I know it will hurt to find out that bacon, shrimp, lobster, crab, and catfish are on the unclean list.

As outlined primarily in Genesis 1:29 (no sin), Genesis 3:18-19 (after the introduction of sin), and Genesis 9:3 (as the result of mass sin), God's foods include nuts/seeds, fruits, oils, grains, legumes, vegetables, dairy, and animal proteins. God's diet plan is simply to eat His created and prescribed foods in moderate quantities.

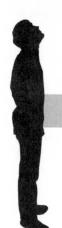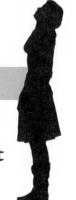

Chapter 18

Seven Practical Dietary Suggestions for Reaching Your Ideal Body Weight

Don't think that overeating and excess weight is solely a consequence of your lack of self-discipline. The body will force you to breathe whether you want to or not. Breathing is not an issue of self-discipline when your body is in need of oxygen. Similarly, if your body is lacking nutrients it will create cravings that you cannot resist.

But you must eat the things God calls food in order to do away with these incessant cravings for nutrients and the weight gain they can cause. These ravenous cravings tend to send us into binges on substances that are anything but healthy, anything but what God wants us to put in our bodies.

Relative to reaching your ideal body weight, the problem with attempting to satisfy nutrient cravings with unhealthy substances is that those nutrient requirements may never be satisfied. It is possible for you to eat 5,000 to 10,000 calories per day of junk non-foods and never escape the feeling of hunger.

It really doesn't matter how much you eat. If your body has not received the nutrients it needs, whether due to the quality or quantity of what you are eating, it will continue to call out for food. Of course, all along the way, your waistline is ever-expanding as it converts all those extra calories into fat.

For someone who is only willing to 'exercise the weight off', and unwilling to improve their diets, this points to another reason why a focused exercise program is not the healthy solution to reaching and maintaining one's ideal body weight. You can't out exercise an unhealthy diet for long. If anything, an exercise program will create more nutrient demands on your body than ever before.

To 'exercise through a bad diet', whether or not it helps you keep most of the fat off for a while, will actually work over time to decrease your general health as your body becomes more and more depleted of nutrients. You may win the battle today but you will eventually lose the war, falling off the wagon, or exercise program as the case may be. Your body is much like an automobile in the sense that it can't keep running well for long without good gas and good oil.

There are two things we need to consider here. One, when you experience cravings for nutrients, you need to seek out healthy sources for those nutrients. A craving for B-vitamins can be satisfied with grilled chicken instead of fried chicken. A craving for Omega-3 oil/fat can be satisfied with oil-rich fish instead of seeking out fats from unhealthy sources like fried foods, pastries, and ice-cream. But this is more reactive than proactive, requiring lots of self-discipline, which brings us to the second consideration.

Don't get me wrong, self-discipline, or self-control, is part of the fruit of the Spirit, a by-product of spiritual conditioning. It is something you need to have to be successful in reaching your ideal body weight. But I think it is wise to reduce the number of tempting moments you will experience by seeking to be proactive, not reactive, in your dietary practices.

It is better to be proactive rather than reactive regarding your nutrient needs. How do you achieve this? You provide your body with the nutrients it needs before it needs them. This can be done by introducing certain foods into your diet on a daily, consistent basis. These are foods that provide you with a consistent flow of the types of nutrients that will effectively ward off the most potentially dangerous cravings.

Suggestion 1: Omega-3 Essential Fatty Acids

I would suggest to you that the most important nutrient issue in our modern world, the nutrient deficiency that may be the most responsible for your inability to reach your ideal body weight, is a lack of essential fatty acids. I would specifically narrow this down to a deficiency of the Omega-3 essential fatty acid.

So step one in your proactive assault on meeting your nutrient needs, before experiencing cravings for that nutrient that send you down an unhealthy eating path, is to start each day with one to two tablespoons of Omega-3 essential fatty acids. My preferred source for this nutrient is cod-liver oil.

You will want to take this in liquid form. The pill form will have you belching and tasting the cod-liver oil all day long. While the liquid form, in my experience, doesn't have that effect. Also, the coating on most capsules is a pork product, not God-approved for consumption.

Straight cod-liver oil is pretty nasty stuff taste-wise. I use a brand that adds mint. The mint does a great job of making the cod-liver oil easy to take. But don't get the brands that add more than just mint. There are brands out there that are only half cod-liver oil. The rest are additives that make the product literally taste like candy, leaving you with only half of the cod-liver oil for your money and some unhealthy ingredients.

Another good source of Omega-3 essential fatty acids would be flaxseed oil, which has the added benefit of also containing Omega-6 and Omega-9 essential fatty acids. The greater deficiency issue for most of us will revolve around the Omega-3, but getting some extra Omega-6 and Omega-9 certainly won't hurt anything either. I sometimes alternate a bottle of cod-liver oil with a bottle of flaxseed oil.

For those of you who are including foods like oil-rich fish in your diet on a consistent basis, you may find that this additional supplementation is unnecessary. But for most of us, maybe even for all of us as a consistent and reliable safety-net if nothing else, we need to supplement our diets to get the Omega-3 our bodies require.

What you will find as you begin introducing the Omega-3 essential fatty acids into your diet each day is that you desire less food. You will also find that it is easier to make healthier choices as well. This is something you will experience with very little need for self-discipline.

I have always craved milk my whole life, drinking it to excessive, fat-gaining levels. But I have noticed that when I include Omega-3 oils in my diet each day that I have very few cravings for milk. That is not to say that milk is unhealthy, but that several glasses of milk every day, especially if consumed along with cookies or cake, will ensure a broad waistline.

Without Omega-3 oils in my diet, my excessive cravings for milk were most likely caused by my body's cravings for fat, Omega-3 specifically. Unfortunately, grain-fed cows do not produce the Omega-3 rich milk that grass-fed cows do. So for me, without cod-liver oil, I was living, like most people, with a life-long deficiency of Omega-3 essential fatty acids.

Our bodies will keep craving various sources of fat anytime there is a deficiency of Omega-3 essential fatty acids in the diet. And for the average American, that nutrient deficiency and craving has existed their entire lives. Is it any wonder that each generation is getting further and further away from their ideal body weight?

Don't even think about trying to reach your ideal body weight without introducing Omega-3 essential fatty acids into your diet. It may very well prove to be the difference between success and failure for you. That is just how important it is.

Suggestion 2: Daily Fruit & Salad

The second addition I would suggest you to make is to ensure you begin introducing life-force foods into your diet by eating at least one piece of fruit and one salad every day. The difference in your sense of well-being (energy, alertness, lack of food cravings, etc.) between a day that includes fruit and salad (raw, uncooked, life-force foods) and a day that does not will be quite noticeable.

Arguably the second greatest nutrient deficiency in our modern diet is a lack of live food. Even healthy cooked foods, as full of nutrients as they may be, lack a life-force, for lack of a better term, that can only come from raw, uncooked foods.

You will especially notice an ever-increasing sense of well-being after implementing this practice for a week or two. It is after this period of time that the fibrous content of these life-force foods will have begun to have a powerful effect on the cleansing of your body of slow-moving and impacted toxins that have built up in your intestinal tract and colon.

I would also suggest eating an apple or orange, for example, 30 minutes before each meal. This is a quick way to get hunger-curbing fiber and nutrients into your body before beginning the meal. It is said that we need to eat slowly because it can take the stomach up to 20 minutes to tell our minds that it is full. Within that extra 20 minutes we might end up eating twice as much food as we really needed. This little fruit trick will help with that issue.

Also, eating fluid-rich fruit 30 minutes before each meal will help ensure you don't need to drink any fluids during your meals, not even water. This is important for two reasons. One, drinking fluids during a meal can work to dilute the digestive juices in your stomach, which could contribute to acid-reflux, gas, and ineffective extraction of nutrients from the food. Also, you may like certain fluids, unhealthy ones, with certain foods and junk non-foods. You may tend to prefer soda or sugary tea over water with your meals (my tendency). By simply eliminating fluids from the meal altogether that issue may go away for you. This technique works great for me.

I also find that my stomach shrinks significantly, on the inside, when I move away from drinking fluids with my meals. In a typical meal it is easy to drink as much, or two to three times as much, in fluid volume, than the volume of food you might consume. Your waist-size will drop very quickly within a matter of weeks from this one simple technique alone, no fat loss necessary.

Even at your ideal body weight you can vary your average waist-size by up to 2 to 3 inches depending on whether or not you 'stretch' your inner stomach by taking in too much volume during meals. Who hasn't experienced that, at least temporarily, from even a single gluttonous outing?

And with a smaller inner stomach will also come less frequent hunger pangs and a lesser volume of food consumed. There seems to be a correlation between the size of our inner stomachs and the frequency of hunger pangs we experience (smaller stomach equals fewer hunger pangs), and of course, the volume of food we can consume. That is what lap-band and other related types of surgeries are all about. Save your money and the damage those procedures will do to your body, and shrink your stomach yourself by not drinking fluids with your meals.

There are even further benefits to excluding fluids from your meals. I tend to be very sensitive to the energy drain that comes from eating. I have noticed that this energy drain is greatly reduced or eliminated when I omit fluids from my meals. This will be especially valuable to those of you who tend to experience the after-lunch energy drop that leads you to the coffee pot.

Also, without the extra volume of fluids during a meal, I never reach that 'stuffed' feeling. It is great to eat in such a way as to not have to experience that kind of discomfort on a daily basis, which was the case with me as someone with tendencies towards overeating.

And I think I tend to eat less food as well when I don't include fluids with my meals. This may be because the density of nutrition per unit volume consumed is greatly increased when only solids are consumed at a meal. The practice of omitting fluids from my meals has absolutely and dramatically improved my diet experience and results.

By the way, whether fruit or something else, it is sometimes good to 'eat before you eat.' If you know you will be in an environment that will test your commitment to dietary holiness, it might be a good idea to take the edge off your hunger with a snack beforehand.

You might be concerned that you normally get thirsty during a meal, requiring fluids. There are only three reasons why you might get thirsty during a meal.

1) You have not kept well-hydrated with water and fruit between meals
2) You are eating unhealthy things
3) You are eating too much

Relative to eating too much, I would suggest, as a rule of thumb, that you not eat past the point of reaching thirst. I am not saying that you should keep eating <u>until</u> you become thirsty, because that may mean you consume too much food at times.

You can actually use this to test whether something is healthy for you or not in some cases. For example, I recently purchased a granola-based health/snack bar. The package included two small, thin bars. Although I had been drinking water throughout the day up until this point, fully hydrated, I was dying of thirst by the time I finished the first bar.

Regardless of what the 'nutrition facts' say, or the summary of health benefits noted on the packet, my body told me that this concoction was not healthy for my body. That granola-based health/snack bar might be less unhealthy for me than a donut, but I still need to go with better alternatives for a snack than that.

Here's another example, a fruit drink. Surely a drink made by blending a few pieces of fruit in a blender should be just as healthy as eating them as solids. It is all the same, so it would seem. Well, maybe not. I find that I am extremely thirsty after drinking a fruit drink, while I feel very hydrated after eating a piece of fruit. What is the difference?

I think the difference comes in the digestive process. The first step in the digestive process is the release of digestive juices in the mouth while chewing the food. When we drink a fruit drink, unless we drink it very slowly and swish it about a bit before swallowing, we substantially bypass the first step in the digestive process, the release of digestive juices in the mouth that occurs while chewing the food. There may be other digestive processes further down the line that are set in motion in the body by the act of chewing as well.

Always remember, anytime we modify the foods God created for us, even modifying to the limited extent of using a blender, we may find ourselves on shaky ground from a health standpoint. As much as possible, don't get fancy with appliances and various processes when it comes to God's foods. You don't need to 'blend' or 'juice'. These are man-made gimmicks and products that will do more to financially benefit their creators than to physically benefit you. You will get plenty of nutrients from the healthy foods you can eat in their God-made forms, so save your money and your countertop space.

I sometimes find that a piece of fruit and a handful of nuts was all my body needed to start with. You aren't obligated to sit down to a seven course meal every meal, or even every day. As your body begins to gain ground, filling up on the nutrients it needs (going from a deficiency to a surplus), you will find yourself eating smaller meals and less frequent meals. Just listen to your body. God designed your body to not lead you astray, but directly to your ideal body weight.

Suggestion 3: Ezekiel 4:9 Bread

The third addition I would encourage you to make to your diet is that you eat two pieces of Ezekiel 4:9 bread each day. You will notice a reduction in your body's cravings for carbohydrates through the practice of eating Ezekiel 4:9 bread each day, a significant component of your effort to reach your ideal body weight. This bread is formulated after the bread recipe that God gave Ezekiel in Ezekiel 4:9. I guess we shouldn't be surprised to learn that this bread is extremely healthy for us. You will typically find this bread in the freezer within the health-food section of a grocery store (if they have a health-food section) or at a health-food store.

It's no secret that junk-carbs like white breads and crackers will cause weight-gain, providing very little in the way of nutrition on top of that. Ezekiel 4:9 bread will help to reduce your draw towards unhealthy carbohydrates. I am not going to try to explain why Ezekiel 4:9 is so healthy. Just trust me on this one, or if interested, do your own research on it.

I often eat two pieces of Ezekiel 4:9 bread with my salad. I also like two toasted pieces of Ezekiel 4:9 bread with honey and strawberries for breakfast, quite delicious with a glass of milk. And a turkey sandwich is also a good way to get some Ezekiel 4:9 bread into your diet.

Suggestion 4: Eggs

The fourth addition I would suggest you make to your diet is eggs. Eat two or more eggs several times each week, more often would be even better. I eat up to 20 eggs a week at times.

I can hear your gasp after reading this recommendation. The health 'experts' say that the fat in the eggs will make you fat, that low-fat is the way to reach your ideal body weight. The health 'experts' also say that the cholesterol in eggs will collect in your bloodstream.

Before I address these inaccurate scientific claims, let's first look to God's Word regarding eggs. We could start and stop with God's Word for that matter, but maybe you are like me and enjoy the science of it all. Are you surprised to know that God would speak specifically about eggs?

"... ask, and it shall be given you; seek, and ye shall find; knock and it shall be opened to you. For every one that asketh receiveth; and he that seeketh findeth; and to him that knocketh it shall be opened. If a son shall ask bread of any of you that is a father, will he give him a stone? Or if he ask a fish, will he for a fish give him a serpent? Or if he shall ask an egg, will he offer him a scorpion? If ye then, being evil, know how to give good gifts unto your children; how much more shall your heavenly Father give the Holy Spirit to them that ask him?" (Luke 11:9-13, KJV)

Prayer will be an important part of your journey towards reaching your ideal body weight as mentioned earlier. As this passage points out, God is anxious to bless you with good things as you might request through prayer. God desires that you live out your life at your ideal body weight, full of energy, vitality, and a zest for living the life He wants for you.

This passage also addresses diet. God often addresses very practical life issues within what we might tend to view as the more spiritual lessons (prayer). In this passage, God outlines dietary examples of bad things and good things; stone (bad) verses bread (good), serpent (bad) verses fish (good), and scorpion (bad) verses egg (good).

So there you have it. God settled the 'egg debate' for us about two thousand years ago. Eggs are good for you. Not that you need to understand the science of why eggs are so good for you, but I will give you some insight into that just the same.

I once conducted a nutritional study of over 30 nutrients. I wanted to determine the primary food sources for each. My analysis showed me the two most nutrient dense foods on the planet. One of those two foods was the 'incredible, edible egg.' The egg is a major source of literally half of every nutrient type that I studied. I will tell you about the other nutrient dense food soon.

But won't the fat in the eggs make me fat? No. The fat in a healthy food is much less likely to be converted to fat in your body than refined sugars and refined flours, for example. Your body needs healthy fats. 50% of your brain is made up of fat. Every cell in your body is wrapped in a membrane of fat. Fat is essential to good health. Fat will be essential to you reaching your ideal body weight. So don't even think about going on a low-fat diet.

But won't the cholesterol in the eggs increase the bad cholesterol in my bloodstream? No. Once again, it will be refined sugars and refined flours that will work to form bad cholesterol in your bloodstream. The cholesterol in healthy foods will not result in the formation of bad cholesterol in the bloodstream. And further regarding the phobia of eating cholesterol rich foods, cholesterol is essential to hormone production in the body. The statement that you are only as healthy as your hormones is a fairly accurate one.

Eating eggs will go a long way towards providing your body with the total nutrition it needs, effectively working to eliminate food cravings from your daily life. This will help you reach your ideal body weight.

Suggestion 5: Dark Green Leafy Vegetables

The fifth addition I suggest you make to your diet is dark green leafy vegetables. Eat a serving or two of cooked dark green leafy vegetables several times a week, more often would be even better. I am differentiating cooked dark green leafy vegetables from the salad I recommended earlier.

During the discussion of eggs I mentioned an analysis I had performed that showed me the two most nutrient dense foods on the planet. You guessed it. The second of those two super-foods is dark green leafy vegetables like spinach or collard greens.

Of the over 30 nutrients that I studied, dark green leafy vegetables were cited as a significant source of over half of them. The consumption of dark green leafy vegetables is an essential component in your journey towards your ideal body weight.

By the way, for those of you who tend to crave chocolate, dark green leafy vegetables may help to curb or eliminate those cravings. It is my understanding that chocolate cravings are primarily an issue of magnesium deficiency. Dark green leafy vegetables are an excellent source of magnesium. Women are typically known to crave chocolate more than men. There is a reason for that. The female body, pound for pound, burns up / requires more magnesium than the male body.

Suggestion 6: Eliminate Caffeine

The sixth recommendation I have for you is to eliminate caffeine from your life. I know this sounds like an impossible request to many. But with

spiritual conditioning and a righteou[...]
will not be impossible for you.

Once you wean yourself off of caffeine, y[...]
a depth of rest at night like you have never e[...]
will begin to develop an ever-increasing sense of v[...]
know has come from eliminating caffeine from your lif[...]
towards healthy foods will increase almost unconsciously.

In my observation and experience, the tendency to eat u[...]
things increases in direct proportion to an increase in fluids like [...]
and soda. For me, I would tend to favor coffee breaks over fruit brea[...]
literally meaning that if I am on coffee I will tend to not eat fruit. I would
often use coffee to curb my hunger, thereby furthering my nutritional
and energy crisis. This can only lead to weight gain.

Soda, a very bad fluid, makes me want unhealthy non-foods to go
with it. I never want grilled meats and vegetables with soda. I want fried
foods and chips with soda.

If you will follow through with the elimination of caffeine from your
diet your health and body weight will improve significantly. There will
be no doubt in your mind that your caffeine addiction has hindered you
from reaching your ideal body weight.

I will continue with a more detailed discussion regarding the effect
of caffeine on reaching your ideal body weight in the next chapter.

Suggestion 7: Water

The seventh recommendation I would make for you is that you simply
keep a bottle of water with you at all times, most especially during the
healing crisis phase. I will talk more about the healing crisis in the next
chapter.

As you give your dietary practices over to God your body will begin
to dump toxins into your bloodstream and intestinal tract at an alarming
rate, part of the healing crisis. Water will be an important component in
that process. Expect to be very thirsty for water and expect a lot of trips

ng God's Weigh. This
ıd that you are well on
you will find that the
ill hold in the form of

self to drink a certain
for water will come
his book concerning
ɔu only need to work
rced. Just cooperate
ıdy and you will do

s motivation leading the way, this
ou will begin to experience
perienced before. You
tality that you will
And your draw
nhealthy
coffee
s,

In summary, include the following items in your diet each day ...

1) One to two tablespoons of cod-liver oil or flaxseed oil (Omega-3 source)
2) One piece of fruit and one salad (life-force and fiber)
3) Two pieces of Ezekiel 4:9 bread (reduced carb cravings)
4) Eat eggs several times each week, if not daily (nutrient-dense)
5) Eat dark green leafy vegetables several times each week, if not daily (nutrient-dense)
6) Eliminate caffeine (removal of chemically-induced stress and nutrient drain)
7) Keep a bottle of water with you at all times (detoxification process)

I am not saying that a daily diet of these things along with half of a gallon of ice-cream, a family-size bag of chips, and 2 liters of caffeine-free soda will enable you to reach your ideal body weight. But what you will find is that as you commit yourself to successfully including these food-types into your diet each day (proactive nutrient supply) your cravings for ice-cream, chips, and soda will slowly and strangely begin to disappear.

In its place you will find yourself eating healthy meats, vegetables, fruits, and nuts/seeds, and drinking more water. This new and improved way of eating that you will begin to experience will require much less self-discipline than a more reactive dietary strategy, and will help pave the way to reaching your ideal body weight.

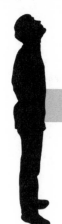
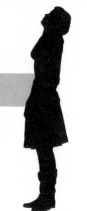

Chapter 19

The Effect of Caffeine on Reaching Your Ideal Body Weight

Caffeine creates a chemically-induced emergency response in the body. This is what leads to that surge of energy you feel. This emergency response is basically the same hormonal response/process that is set in motion when a real emergency springs upon you, say like seeing a lion standing in the doorway of your home.

No matter how fatigued you might have felt before you saw that lion you will have an incredible surge of energy afterwards. When you see that lion the chemical and hormonal response that is activated involves the adrenals, the production of the adrenal hormone cortisol, and the release of glucose into the bloodstream. Caffeine enacts these same elements. It is that release of glucose into the bloodstream that gives you the sense of energy you feel.

So what is the problem with this? How does caffeine negatively impact your body weight? I will answer those questions for you right now.

I know what it means to reach that point when I lose even that temporary surge of energy that should come from caffeine. This is an indication of what some call chronic fatigue. Chronic fatigue occurs gradually over time as our bodies become more and more worn out from the abuses we have put them through.

'Worn out' is really not an accurate statement. Your body isn't worn out, although it may feel that way. What you are experiencing is your body's attempt at survival, despite your best attempts to kill it. When you have pushed too far for too long, God has designed your body to rev-down, whether you and your circumstances like it or not.

What is really happening is that your central nervous system and hypothalamus-pituitary-thyroid control centers are directing your body to get some rest, in a nutshell. This is brought about by hormonal adjustments that work to slow the body down.

There is an epidemic of hypothyroidism (slowed thyroid function) diagnosis today that is based on a lack of understanding of how the body works in this way. The problem is not a slowed thyroid and the corresponding reduction in thyroid hormones that leads to a slowed metabolism. The truth is quite to the contrary. This 'hypothyroidism' is the body's 'answer' to an unhealthy diet and a lack of rest. The 'problem' is that we continue to refuse to live Godly lives regarding diet and rest.

The body is trying to get some rest for survival. The body wants, and has commanded in effect, that the production of hormones from the thyroid gland be reduced in an effort to slow itself down. The body is trying to force you to conserve energy and to get some rest. Taking thyroid hormone supplements, as prescribed after a diagnosis of hypothyroidism, will only work to make your condition worse. As well-meaning as the doctors, nurses, and administrators may be, man's wisdom is predominately what you will find in the healthcare industry. This is a perfect example.

It's our fleshly desire to 'have it all' that keeps the healthcare industry booming. We want our ideal body weight and we want our soda, milkshakes, and cookies too. And we are willing to take medications to increase our metabolism to get it. Unfortunately, even the misguided willingness to sacrifice our future health for a temporal pleasure, in the end, doesn't get us to our ideal body weight and only leaves us worse off than before we started. This will always be the pattern and consequence of man's way; of not looking to God for the solution to life's challenges.

This same principle applies to caffeine. We want enough energy to be productive at work. We want enough energy to get through some 'exercise program.' We also want our soda, milkshakes, and cookies. And we don't want to live in such a way as to get the rest we need (a sober life). So what do we do? We self-prescribe caffeine to save the day. With both thyroid hormone supplementation and caffeine, you may win the battle (not much of a victory if at all) but you will lose the war (you will be less likely to reach your ideal body weight and your health will be negatively affected).

Caffeine takes a loan out against tomorrow's health to get you through today. It is much like running your car at 120 mph everywhere you go. You may get places quicker and get more done today, but you will eventually begin to have more mechanical problems, and your vehicle's total potential miles will be reduced.

The necessity for the abuse of caffeine comes primarily in the form of refusing to listen to your body's signals. Your body is intelligently designed, by God almighty Himself, and it is screaming for attention. Your body is literally calling out to you to seek Godly wisdom, whether you recognize it or not. Your journey to your ideal body weight will require that you get in sync with how God made your body, listening and responding to what your body tells you, not forcing your body to function through the chemically-induced emergency response brought on by caffeine.

I realize that this all sounds logical right up until about 10:00AM on Monday morning. You are in your office feeling groggy (your body telling you that your diet and rest is not adequate) and you have work that must be completed for your presentation to upper management at noon. Your body is telling you that it needs rest, that your diet and rest have not been adequate to provide you with an energetic, productive day.

What do you do? In the short-run there may not be much you can do. The best recommendation I can give you might be to take a week off from work as soon as it can be scheduled. Your goal for that week is to wean yourself off caffeine and fully devote yourself to rest. In the long-run, as promoted by this book, look to God for wisdom and walk in obedience to His directives for living in all areas, certainly to include diet and rest.

That cup of coffee and donut you eat to keep you going, in conjunction with your body's attempt to slow down your metabolism, brings about inevitable weight gain and poor overall health. The elimination of caffeine from your diet will prove to be an important component of your journey towards your ideal body weight.

Many people are living their lives in a state of chronic fatigue. At some point you just can't keep 'going to the well' and expecting the supply to be there. The daily consumption of caffeine, especially when used to compensate for your lack of energy due to a poor diet and lack of rest, revs the body up when the body wants/needs to slow down. Common sense will tell you that putting your body into such an extreme situation will only wear it out further by the day. Your body is calling for rest. But rather than getting that rest, many people are throwing their bodies into a chemically-induced emergency with caffeinated coffee, soda, or tea.

Although weight loss is not dependent upon an exercise program as discussed earlier, I do believe that physical activity is an important part of good health and an important part of a happy, productive life. God made us to be physically active. Ultimately, physical activity will play an important role in expediting your journey to your ideal body weight. But if you are chronically fatigued then a physically active lifestyle isn't going to happen. And overweight or not, a chronically fatigued life is no life at all.

The flow of caffeine during the day will also negatively impact the quality of your sleep at night. This is because the work of caffeine in the body tends toward chronically higher cortisol levels. Cortisol is often referred to as the 'stress hormone'. God designed the body to have higher levels of cortisol first thing in the morning (to get you going) and lower levels in the evening (to prepare you for rest). As mentioned earlier, cortisol is also part of our body's emergency response system.

Caffeine consumption works toward producing higher cortisol levels in the evening, impairing your body's ability to get the depth of restful sleep it needs. You can see the viscous cycle that this creates. Being off caffeine, if I have so much as one 12-ounce soda during the day, even as early as noon, I can tell that the quality of my sleep that night has been negatively impacted.

The body is designed to cope with infrequent stresses, not the type of chronic stress that caffeine creates in the body day after day. Also, at least in the corporate office environment, the hormonal response that occurs has little to no relief in the way of 'burning off' the glucose that has been dumped into the bloodstream.

Why is it important to know this regarding reaching your ideal body weight? The glucose that is dumped into the bloodstream for the purpose of immediate energy comes from the liver. Unfortunately, any leftover glucose that is not utilized does not go back to the liver. This excess glucose will be stored on the body in the form of fat, unless you go run a mile after each cup of coffee.

In more primitive times, the body's response to seeing a lion would have been activated less frequently. And the physical response (running and hiding) would have rebalanced the body's hormone levels subsequent to the emergency, and burned up the extra glucose in the bloodstream.

This is unlike what we experience through the daily consumption of caffeine as we continue to sit at our computers after we drink our cup of coffee. And it is not an infrequent occurrence either. Our daily consumption of caffeine is often a continuous flow of caffeine, day in and day out, with coffee in the morning and afternoon, soda at lunch, and tea at dinner.

When I was growing up I did not realize that tea had caffeine in it. My parents didn't know either, at least they never warned me otherwise. In any event, I would routinely eat a sleeve of saltine crackers along with a tall glass of tea in the evenings before bed. It would take me two hours to fall asleep. I thought I had insomnia.

The more caffeine you consume the more food cravings you may have. The chemically-induced emergency response caused by caffeine uses up a lot of nutrients, which the body demands be replenished. That is where the food cravings come from.

Food cravings related to caffeine consumption also come from caffeine's effect on quality sleep. Quality sleep is a critical component of rest, good health, and body weight control.

Without the rest it needs, the body will ultimately call for more carbohydrates. This is true for two reasons. One, a fatigued body burns up large quantities of B-vitamins and other nutrients, which it often seeks to replenish through carbohydrate consumption. Unfortunately, the types of carbohydrates we tend to gravitate towards are refined carbohydrates, lacking the nutrients our bodies are craving. Unless we get these nutrient cravings satisfied by way of a healthy carbohydrate source, we can find ourselves consuming refined carbohydrates throughout the day, taking in an excessive volume of calories along the way. And two, a fatigued body tends to seek to be 'perked up' with the quick energy that carbohydrates can provide.

So here you are. Your metabolism is slowing down due to fatigue and your carbohydrate cravings are increasing, the perfect formula for weight gain. This is why good rest is a critical component of losing fat and reaching your ideal body weight. I have often wondered which is more important for weight loss, a good diet or good rest. Both are extremely important.

It would be helpful for me to explain the 'healing crisis' at this point. The healing crisis, as it is sometimes referred, involves the fact that you may feel worse while you are getting better. Getting off caffeine provides the perfect example.

You have probably attempted to get off caffeine at some point in your life. And maybe you quit cold-turkey, all at once. With the exception of some fatigue, you might have weathered the first day of that process without too much difficulty. But then came day two, and the caffeine withdrawal headache. Man, oh man, did it hurt. This is an example of the healing crisis. You feel worse on your way to getting better.

I might suggest slowly weaning yourself off caffeine in an effort to avoid the cold-turkey induced, caffeine withdrawal headache. What has worked for me is to reduce my caffeine intake down to zero gradually over several days, say from 4 cups of coffee to 3 to 2 to 1 to 0. And on the day that I reached 'zero', if I should happen to feel a caffeine withdrawal headache coming on, I needed only to drink about 4 ounces of coffee to knock it out. I might have had to drink another 4-ounce coffee later in the day as well. And then, as my body more deeply adjusted to the absence of caffeine, I might have felt a dull head-ache come on every two to three days for another week or two. Again, drinking a 4-ounce coffee each time took care of those few remaining episodes.

You could also try bypassing the gradual reduction in coffee intake and go straight to taking small shots of coffee (4 ounces at a time) each time a caffeine withdrawal headache might develop.

Once off the caffeine, you will also experience another symptom. I suppose this symptom is related to your body realizing it can finally get some much needed rest. You may find yourself doing some of the most exaggerated stretching and deep yawns of your life. It will be very obvious to you because your normal intake of caffeine has kept your body from ever reaching this point of deep relaxation.

It is worth noting that an expedited release and elimination of built-up toxins from the body can be expected when you begin to eat as God directs, especially during the first month. That is good news. The bad news is that the acute elimination of toxins during this period can, and in a sense does, overload the body.

Much like the caffeine withdrawal headache, the net result is that you may feel a bit sickly at times along the way. But it won't be a sickness like a cold or flu, although it can feel similar in its own way. One simple example of a symptom that you might experience will be fatigue. As we discussed earlier, if your body needs rest to recuperate and/or in order to redirect more energy to the process of toxin elimination, it may work to slow you down at times (make you feel tired).

You could also experience chills, finding that you have to wear a jacket or sweater when everyone else seems okay without one. What is happening is that the body is diverting energy and warmth away from the exterior of your body in favor of application to the interior of your body to help with the process of toxin elimination.

Listen to your body during these times and do what it's telling you to do, rest and keep warm. Unfortunately, you will have to travel through the valley of the healing crisis before getting to the hilltop of vitality on the other side.

The healing crisis will occur in ever-decreasing intensity and frequency as your health improves over time. You may experience episodes of the healing crisis for several weeks, several months, or even up to a year. Your level of physical health before you begin God's diet will determine just how long it will take for your body to right itself chemically and hormonally. Be patient in knowing that you are walking in obedience to God's Word, that you have given rightful ownership of your body back to Him.

Before moving on, I want to mention something about allergies and caffeine. Each Fall I am susceptible to an allergic response to something in the environment, whether mold, ragweed, or whatever. This allergic response includes some of the typical watery eyes and sneezing types of symptoms, but it goes much further than that for me.

This allergic response includes a tendency for me to need to withdraw from people. I just want to crawl in a cave and be left alone. I call it my Fall Funk. I don't fully understand what is happening on a physiological level other than to say that the impact of some Fall allergen is so significant that I can be outgoing in the Spring and be a recluse in the Fall.

The only thing that has seemed to divert this allergic response, this Fall Funk, has been getting off caffeine. It may simply be that the deep rest that caffeine-free living allows, in conjunction with doing away with the nutrient-depleting tendencies of caffeine, equips and strengthens my body in its resilience against the onslaught of allergens. But whatever it is, I will tell you that getting off caffeine changed my life in a major way with respect to allergies and the Fall Funk I would normally experience.

Caffeine may also negatively affect your blood-pressure. Coffee and sodas are more difficult for the kidneys to process than water. My mother-in-law had cysts on her breasts that her doctor attributed to caffeine consumption. We may never know all of the negative effects of caffeine on the body, but I would expect continued study to reveal more and more that caffeine works as a degenerative agent in our bodies.

If you are serious about getting healthy and reaching your ideal body weight, then get off the caffeine. And know this. After a month or so you will be pleasantly surprised to discover that the thought of consuming liquid black sludge like coffee and soda is very unappealing. You will wonder what ever got you to liking that stuff to begin with.

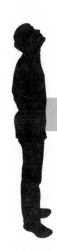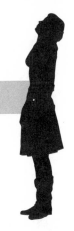

Chapter 20

The Effect of Stress on Reaching Your Ideal Body Weight

Stress can have a significantly negative impact on your body's ability to reach its ideal body weight. For some, stress works to whittle them down to a bag of bones, to below their ideal body weight. But I would contend that for most of us, stress has a tendency to cause weight gain. The Biblical principles concerning diet and health, and life in general, will bring both types of people back to their ideal body weights.

But even for those who may experience overall weight gain due to the impact of stress on their bodies and minds, they will typically experience a whittling down of their musculature and overall health as well. I did a health analysis on someone who had lost a net 3 pounds over the previous five years, per the scale. On the surface this might seem to be a positive report, but upon further analysis I was able to determine that he had lost 15 pounds of muscle during that period.

So what actually happened was that he had lost 15 pounds of muscle and gained 12 pounds of fat, for a net loss of 3 pounds on the scale. The truth of the matter is that his body had not improved my 3 pounds but had changed by a negative 27 pounds (15 pounds of muscle lost and 12 pounds of fat gained).

Stress creates a chemical and hormonal response in your body that is designed to help you cope with that stress. This is a good thing that your body is designed to do for you. But God did not intend for you to live in the state of chronic stress that most of us have found ourselves in today.

While the effect of infrequent stress will have little to no negative effect on your body weight, chronic stress will. The stress-response process ultimately works to dump glucose out of the liver and into the bloodstream for the immediate energy required to respond to the stress/emergency. In a more primitive, less modern time and place, this extra glucose would have been burned up as you ran from a lion, hurried through the woods, or wrestled with an adversary.

But what are you typically doing when stress at work comes upon you? You are sitting in a conference room or at your desk. You aren't in a situation or involved in an activity that will burn off all of that glucose that has been dumped into your bloodstream in response to your view of something as stressful or an emergency. So what happens to all that glucose that has been dumped into your bloodstream?

Whatever glucose is leftover after the nervous energy that you might expend tapping your pencil on the table or shuffling your feet, unfortunately, is not returned to the liver. This leftover glucose is converted to fat. So unless you get up and go for a quick jog right after that stressful event you may very well experience some fat accumulation from it. That sure puts a whole new perspective on career choice and stress.

Also, stress provides the opportunity to increase body weight through the nutritional demands that it creates. The chemical and hormonal response that stress induces in your body burns up a lot of nutrients as your body works to get itself into emergency response mode, ready for action. This will inevitably lead to food cravings as your body lets you know that those nutrients need to be replaced. And the nutrients that need to be replaced will include the B-vitamins, which will lead to carbohydrate cravings specifically.

If you don't replenish the nutrients used up during a stressful event with healthy food you will most likely end up consuming extra calories that are later converted to fat. The more frequent the occurrence of these nutrient-depleting, stressful events the more often your body will call upon you to replenish those nutrients and the more often will be your opportunity to eat too much food and/or unhealthy non-foods. These are opportunities for fat gain, and muscle loss as well.

Eventually your body will respond to this chronic onslaught of stress by trying to get some rest. This comes in the form of a slowed metabolism. Although a slowed metabolism is the best direction for your body's long-term survival, you will not be happy with the added weight gain that may follow.

So relative to reaching your ideal body weight you have a quadruple whammy that can occur from chronic stress...

1) Fat gain from unused blood glucose
2) Fat gain from carbohydrate cravings and/or unhealthy eating following nutrient loss
3) Fat gain from a slowed metabolism
4) Muscle loss

Although the amount of fat gain and muscle loss may occur at a small fraction of an ounce per occurrence, over time, the impact can be significant. Even if this quadruple whammy only resulted in a fat gain and/or muscle loss of 1/8 ounce per day, in a year the net degeneration in body composition would be 2.85 pounds per year (365 days x 1/8 ounce x 1 pound per 16 ounces). That may not be too far from what many middle-aged folks are experiencing, maybe even on the low side at that.

Over twenty years, say from the age of 35 to 55, the total degenerative effect of stress on the body, in this example, would be 57 pounds. Looking back at the example above, this 57 pounds may actually only show up as a net weight gain of 33 pounds on the scale (say 45 pounds of fat gained and 12 pounds of muscle lost). So the situation is much worse than just 33 pounds gained. It will be body composition that reveals the total damage. Although what is reflected on the scale seems bad enough, the true impact of stress and unhealthy eating is even worse.

The chronic stress in your life comes in two forms. One, some of that chronic stress is thrust upon you from the outside modern world. And two, some of that stress comes about by your own choices. In both cases you need to look to God for wisdom, guidance, and strength to overcome the negative effects of stress on your health and on your body weight.

Let's first look at the chronic stresses thrust upon you by the world around you and what you can do about it. I will use a couple of examples of circumstances that can produce chronic stress in our lives, the corporate work environment and the government school system.

Over the past ten to fifteen years the quality of life in the workplace has declined significantly. It has become more demanding. It has become more cold and impersonal. It has become more mechanized and technologically oriented. It has become more demanding of the employee's time. And God is no longer allowed there.

And over the past few years specifically, Corporate America has become a police state with everybody worried that everyone else will report them for one offense or another. The extreme caution exercised regarding every word spoken and every action taken is smothering and stressful.

With the economic decline of recent years the attitude in the corporate environment has become one of 'you are lucky to have a job' and 'if you don't like it we can find someone else.' The attitude of upper management, and all levels of management, is becoming less respectful and more demeaning. You are left wondering who is worse off, the ones who have lost their jobs or the ones left behind to do all the work and deal with this environment.

It is getting harder and harder to find a sense of meaning and purpose in the work available through Corporate America. One radio personality

(Michael Berry), speaking about career and purposeful living, said 'Get out of that cubicle and go do something with your life!!!' How much of your life are you willing to give away, doing something that doesn't mean anything to you, doing things that you had just as soon let someone else do, or doing something that isn't in sync with God's design and purpose for you?

Could the stress you have been experiencing at work be God trying to get your attention as He tries to move you down another path? That was my experience. Year after year, decade after decade, I knew something wasn't right. I even knew that God wanted me to write this book. But I kept rationalizing and suffering my way along year after year. God evidently determined I wasn't going to make the move so he made the move with a series of circumstances that led to the loss of my job that could have only come from His divine handiwork. That job loss is why you are getting to read this book right now.

Just because you have a particular job doesn't mean that it is God's desire/will for you. To the extent you seek God will significantly affect whether you are heading down His path for your life, your own path for your life, or someone else's path for your life (parent's, peer's, spouse's…). In any event, just know that God's plan for your life is better than the one you have been able to work out on your own.

Only God can tell you if it is His voice trying to speak to you to move you in a new direction. I don't want to take on the responsibility of telling someone they should leave their current work environment. But I do want to tell you that living a life and working in an environment/career that God has not intended for the way He made you will create stresses in your life that will lead to muscle loss and fat gain.

It takes a lot of faith to move away from the typical American path, but that may be what is standing between you and a meaningful life. It may be that God wants something better for His people. What is the cost for a lack of faith? Isn't it your very soul, and ultimately, your health and your ideal body weight?

"For whoever desires to save his life will lose it, but whoever loses his life for My sake and the gospel's will save it. For what will it profit a man if he gains the whole world, and loses his own soul? Or what will a man give in exchange for his soul?" (Mark 8:35-37, NKJV, BibleGateway.com)

There is a lot on the line when it comes to your career/job choice, even more than your ideal body weight. Consider this statement from Beth Moore.

"We can live with all manner of tribulation more easily than we can live with purposelessness."
(*Discovering God's Purpose for Your Life*, pg. 12, Beth Moore)

Is the corporate environment good for your spiritual walk? Are you amongst a proud people who draw you away from the things of God? Your choice of career/job should go beyond financial considerations.

"Better to be of a humble spirit with the lowly, than to divide the spoil with the proud." (Proverbs 16:19, NKJV, BibleGateway.com)

It's those 'proud' people who boast of the size of their pocket-books, while trying to ignore the size of their waistlines.

And then we have the government school system as another possible chronic stress in our lives. I intentionally replaced 'public' with 'government' because our modern school system is anything but controlled by the public/community anymore. This is more and more becoming an opportunity for great stress in the lives of the parents and the kids as the practices and philosophies of the government school system seem to be moving further and further away from any resemblance of Biblical wisdom. But we should expect that, since God is no longer allowed there. God may be leading you to seek alternative educational opportunities for your children, whether in the form of private-schooling or homeschooling. To ignore His call on your life in this regard will be a great source of stress for you and your children.

But while you are still in these two environments, you still need to successfully cope with the stress. Two important coping mechanisms, for a lack of a better term, include forgiveness and humility. I will not try to create a thesis within this book on forgiveness and humility, but it is important to note that a lack of forgiveness and a lack of humility (in the workplace, at school, at home, in the community) will significantly increase the stress in your life and its impact on you and your body weight.

You will have numerous, even daily, opportunities that require the application of forgiveness and humility in your life. If you live in unforgiveness and pride, the already stressful events you may experience in the corporate work environment and the government school system will be allowed to maximize their negative impact on you, your health, and your body weight, even working to create more problems and stress.

"Pride goes before destruction, and a haughty spirit before a fall." (Proverbs 16:18, NKJV, BibleGateway.com)

You will also need to spend plenty of time in spiritual conditioning through Bible study, prayer, and worship. Frequent reading of the Psalms will also prove very helpful with coping with stress. It is in the Psalms that we get to see David crying out to God and depending upon Him during stressful times in his life.

"Cast thy burden upon the Lord, and he shall sustain thee…" (Psalm 55:22, KJV)

As you seek to determine God's plan for your life you must except that the battle of faith over fear will inevitably be an important part of that journey. You will need to come to learn that control is an illusion.

Control, even if attainable, will not satisfy. And you must understand that being miserable in your life's work is the most irresponsible thing you can do for you, for your family, for your health, and for your body weight.

You must prepare for stressful circumstances by strengthening your body with Godly wisdom, a healthy diet and good rest being important components of that preparation. Don't forget the body-soul-spirit connection. And don't forget that your body is not your own.

God may be seeking to move you in a more meaningful direction than can be found in the typical corporate work environment. And God may be seeking to move your family in a more positive direction than can be found in the government school system.

You must seek God to determine whether you must cope with or remedy these circumstances in your life. This is especially true if these environments draw you and/or your children towards addictive, unhealthy, ungodly practices, whether in the form of diet or something else as you attempt to escape from the stresses. Maybe instead of living a life that requires constant escapes, God would lead you to living a life that is an escape unto itself.

We also have stresses that are brought upon us by our own immediate choices. An unhealthy diet, for example, results in a chemically-induced stress in your body that works to keep you from your ideal body weight. The entirety of this book addresses this issue.

There may be other choices that we make that are not consistent with God's Word, whether that comes in the form of alcohol and tobacco abuse, staying up late watching television, dishonesty, angry and vengeful thoughts towards others, and a host of selfish, ungodly decisions and actions that are available to us.

When we give into various temptations we will heap mounds of stress upon our lives. This stress will work both directly and indirectly to keep us from our ideal body weight.

I believe that the greatest temptation that faces mankind, and one that impacts our stress levels and fat-storage systems greatly, is the temptation to fear. That is not a typo. The temptation to fear is the greatest temptation we face on a daily, even moment by moment, basis. It may be that giving into the temptation to fear is keeping you from your ideal body weight, because of fear's effect both physically and emotionally.

I know it doesn't make any sense at first glance, but stay with me on this point. The reason for the question mark that is on your face right now is that it makes no sense that anyone would be tempted to fear. It would seem that the only thing anyone should be tempted towards would involve pleasure, fear being the furthest thing from pleasure possible.

I realize no one has ever thought to put 'the temptation to fear' on their top ten list of temptations/desires. When considering the topic of temptation, we normally think of materialism and greed, sexual lust, power and control, and unhealthy eating, for example. But deep down in our gut, in our core and unspoken life beliefs, we often believe that fearing a particular challenge, outcome, or person will keep us more on top of a problem and able to more effectively respond to that problem. I think giving into the temptation to fear is what has caused the greatest chronic, long-term stress in my life, and a host of poor decisions.

Giving into the temptation to fear will cause you to make bad life decisions, to include those that directly and indirectly keep you from reaching your ideal body weight. Giving into this temptation will cause you to be overly stressed by life's challenges. Giving into this temptation will cause your relationships with others, even God, to be sour and stressful. It is no wonder that under the control of this temptation a person finds themselves led to emotional eating (emotionally justified eating), as well as eating to replenish the nutrient drain that the stress has directly caused on the body (physiologically justified eating).

There are times when I am still and quiet that I begin to feel drawn to eat. I am not hungry. I am not necessarily even bored. As I pause and more carefully consider where my draw towards eating is coming from I realize that I desire relief from a dull sense of fear that I can't attach to anything specific. I have to catch myself during those times to remind myself that this is the voice of Satan, and to remind myself of the goodness of God.

I think many people in our modern world live with this dull sense of fear. This is probably why most people live life at such a break-neck, drunken pace. Slowing down allows that dull sense of fear to overtake them. At that point they either need to turn to more activity or some addiction with which to medicate. As a Believer, you don't have to do that. You can turn to God and through Him relinquish that dull sense of fear.

This temptation to fear can come in many specific forms; the temptation to fear losing your job, the temptation to fear that someone won't like you, the temptation to fear that everything won't get done that you think should get done, the temptation to fear the unknowns of moving to another town, the temptation to fear physical harm from criminal attack, the temptation to fear the future because of current political policies and personnel, etc.

I had plenty of opportunities to be tempted to fear in getting this book completed and out to you. This book would not have happened without the revelation that 'I must resist the temptation to fear.' There may be a challenge in your life that you have been unwilling to face and overcome because you have given into the temptation to fear.

Regarding some challenges in life, it may be that there is nothing you can do to change that 'thorn in your side.' But the temptation to fear has kept you from accepting it as something that God wants in your life. Maybe you have been unwilling to trust that God's protection, provision, and path will be sufficient. The opposite of faith will always be fear. And when we give in to the temptation to fear, for many of us, emotional and unhealthy eating is not far behind.

You may believe deep down that it would be irresponsible, not 'adult,' for you to not spend significant time afraid of what might happen in some area of your life. But isn't it the faith of a child that God calls us to? We have bought the lie that we should live by fear in order to be responsible adults.

"And Jesus called a little child unto him, and set him in the midst of them, and said, verily I say unto you, except ye be converted, and become as little children, ye shall not enter into the kingdom of heaven." (Matthew 18:2-3, KJV)

The Kingdom of Heaven is one of faith and peace, not one of fear and turmoil. The Kingdom of Heaven is one of health and ideal body weight, not sickness and obesity. It will take some practice to learn to be 'as little children' when your 'be a grown up' voice tells you that stressing over something is the wise and beneficial thing to do.

In the context of your current objective (reaching your ideal body weight), giving in to the temptation to fear will cause hormonal responses in the body that cause fat-storage and cause nutrient deficiencies that lead to hunger pangs/cravings for more food. And it can also lead to emotional eating on top of that.

Now this isn't to say that there are not things in life that should concern us, that we should make plans regarding, for which we should seek God's direction, and for which we should ultimately seek God's peace concerning. But the temptation to fear of which I am referring comes from Satan to torment us, not to lead us to prayer and planning. That is what you must recognize.

You may be tempted to fear that without certain things in your life you can't be happy. You may be tempted to fear that a life without soda and cookies will be a miserable life. This is Satan's lie. It will be in escaping the clutches of an uncontrolled diet that you will find the life you've always dreamed of.

Learning to recognize the voice of Satan speaking into your life is vital. It is in first recognizing the source of the temptation to fear that we can be empowered to disregard it as nothing but Satan's attempt to derail us and to keep us from God's best in our lives, ideal body weight included. This has been a life-transforming revelation in my life. And I believe this same revelation will be an important part of your journey towards your ideal body weight. A life lived in fear will not be a life that leads to health and ideal body weight.

First recognize the source of the temptation to fear (Satan) and disregard it as such, and if further support is necessary, then take your fears to God in prayer.

"Be anxious for nothing, but in everything by prayer and supplication, with thanksgiving, let your requests be made know to God; and the peace of God, which surpasses all understanding will guard your hearts and minds through Christ Jesus." (Philippians 4:6-7, NKJV, BibleGateway.com)

Remember how much God cares for you, that He will always be there to provide for you and meet your needs.

"Are not two sparrows sold for a farthing? And one of them shall not fall on the ground without your Father. But the very hairs of your head are all numbered. Fear ye not therefore, ye are of more value than many sparrows." (Matthew 10:29-31, KJV)

"Casting all your care upon him; for he careth for you." (I Peter 5:7, KJV)

All of us must learn to stop and wait upon God when we are troubled. You must seek His wisdom and His peace regarding life's challenges. The answer is not in a bowl of ice-cream. It is God who must be your salvation, your defense, your expectation, and your refuge from the storms of life. A bowl of ice-cream is a poor substitute for what God offers.

Looking to God for peace is the way to a life lived with purpose and deep, lasting pleasure. Looking to a bowl of ice-cream to make yourself feel better is the way to a life of pursuing pleasure that ultimately ensures you never have purpose or pleasure in your life, a life the result of which will show its ravages in the form of excess weight on your body.

"Truly my soul silently waits for God; from Him comes my salvation. He only is my rock and my salvation. He is my defense. I shall not be greatly moved. My soul, wait silently for God alone. For my expectation is from Him. Trust in Him at all times, you people. Pour out your heart before Him. God is a refuge for us." (Psalm 62:1,2,5,8, NKJV, BibleGateway.com)

You have got to get this one down sooner or later in life. Will you choose God, purpose, and your ideal body weight or will you choose to give in to Satan's deceptions, the pursuit of pleasure without purpose, and obesity? Choose you this day who you will serve and what type of life you will live.

You may as well give in to God now. He will stay after you until you do. Why not save yourself a lot of time and trouble? Why not end the life of shame that you are living? It doesn't have to be this way. It can end right now. Turn to God and His ways and begin to enjoy the life He wants for you, a life lived out at your ideal body weight.

"... choose you this day whom ye will serve... but as for me and my house, we will serve the Lord." (Joshua 24:15, KJV)

"... I have set before you life and death, blessing and cursing; therefore, choose life..." (Deuteronomy 30:19, KJV)

Resisting the temptation to fear, finding the peace of God through prayer, being reminded that God will always care for you, and choosing purpose (life) over pleasure (death) will help to ensure that you don't have the need to turn to emotional and unhealthy eating to compensate for emotional starvation.

You might be able to control your tendencies towards emotional escape through eating, but you will never be able to escape the physiological needs resulting from the nutrient drain caused by stress. That would be like telling your body to breathe less. It can't be done for any effective length of time at all.

Another source of stress is a lack of rest. I sometimes believe that proper rest is more important than a proper diet relative to reaching your ideal body weight. The world says the proper order is exercise – diet – rest. I would contend that the proper order may be rest – diet – exercise.

A lack of good rest throws everything out of whack. Your hormone balance, your metabolism, your energy levels, and your carbohydrate cravings are all negatively affected by a lack of proper rest. You don't have a chance of getting your diet and physical activity down if you are not getting enough rest. This means that you won't have a chance of reaching your ideal body weight.

This is where living a sober life becomes so important. We are called to live a quiet and peaceable life, not a hectic, stimulus-driven, strung-out life. That requires seeking God's direction to achieve a total life makeover. It means conquering addictive and unhealthy behaviors in every area of your life.

While I will contend that getting 8 hours of rest each night will be essential to you reaching your ideal body weight, the total 'rest equation' can be much more complicated than that for those whose entire lives are upside down from how God wants their lives lived. I won't try to attempt to provide you with total life makeover advice in this book, but I do want you to begin seeking God and asking Him what and how you might need to alter your life to His glory.

When considering a good night's sleep, all hours are not the same. I have heard it said that the hours slept before midnight are significantly more restful than the hours slept after midnight. In other words, sleeping from 9PM to 5AM is much more valuable in terms of quality rest than sleeping from 12AM to 8AM, even though the total hours slept may be the same.

This may be true in part because of the increase in cortisol levels that can occur at about 11:00PM if you are still awake. It works like 'clockwork' for me. If I am up at 11:00PM, I get a second wind (cortisol shot) that doesn't allow me to fall asleep until about 1:00AM. This is the body's response to assuming that an emergency must exist if it is still awake at that hour. I would surmise that for those who can still fall asleep during this timeframe that their sleeping cortisol levels are still be higher than had they gotten to sleep earlier, negatively affecting the quality of their sleep. Higher cortisol levels, especially late at night, lead to weight gain.

As a general rule, nothing good happens after 10:00PM, and not just relative to health and body weight. Early to bed, early to rise, makes a man healthy, wealthy, and wise. No truer words have ever been spoken.

Sometimes stress needs to be coped with. Sometimes stress is an indication that you need to move in a new direction. Sometimes stress is an indication that you are giving in to the temptation to fear. Sometimes stress is an indication that you are not making Godly choices in your life, whether with regard to living soberly or getting adequate rest. But in every case, the solution is seeking God's wisdom, power, and direction through Bible study and prayer, then walking in obedience as He would guide you. This will be an important component of your journey to your ideal body weight.

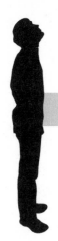
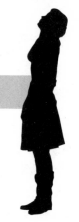

Chapter 21

WWJW ™ – What Would
Jesus Weigh? ™

WWJW – What Would Jesus Weigh? Isn't this an interesting question? It is obviously a spin-off from WWJD – What Would Jesus Do? WWJD became very popular as a tool to remind Believers to consider 'What Would Jesus Do?' when faced with an important decision regarding what to do or say in whatever situation they might find themselves. I think this is a valuable exercise that can be applied to your life every day, multiple times per day at that.

Similarly, I hope that 'WWJW – What Would Jesus Weigh?' might inspire you to approach diet and health the way Jesus approached diet and health. After all, are you not called to be Christ-like?

Although the Bible doesn't tell us how much Jesus' weighed, at least not as far as I am aware, I would submit to you that Jesus would have lived His life at His ideal body weight. How can you know this and what example did Jesus leave to show you the way to your ideal body weight?

I believe Jesus lived His life at His ideal body weight because Jesus lived a perfect life, and a perfect life would have been one walked out in obedience to His Father's commands, in obedience to every component of the wisdom and power of God applicable to diet and health. Therefore, Jesus would have lived His life at His ideal body weight.

I know Jesus would have lived out His life in obedience to His Father's commandments regarding diet and health because He told us to do so as well. And He told us to teach others to do the same.

"Let your light so shine before men, that they may see your good works, and glorify your Father which is in Heaven. Think not that I am come to destroy the law, or the prophets: I am not come to destroy, but to fulfill. For verily I say unto you, till heaven and earth pass, one jot or one tittle shall in no wise pass from the law, till all be fulfilled. Whosoever therefore shall break one of these least commandments, and shall teach men so, he shall be called the least in the kingdom of heaven: but whosoever shall do and teach them, the same shall be called great in the kingdom of heaven." (Matthew 5:16-19, KJV)

These are the words of Jesus Himself. How is it that the Church has been able to convince itself that the dietary directives of God no longer apply to us today after reading a passage like this? Through dietary deception, which involves our fleshly desires, we have been enticed to misinterpret, even modify, Scripture to support our ways. I will cover many of the more common misinterpretations later.

Jesus' purpose on this Earth was not to destroy the law. And I think it is safe for us to assume He was fully aware of Leviticus 11 and Deuteronomy 14 when He said that. As you may recall, in these chapters God spelled out what animal meats should (clean) and should not (unclean) be eaten. The main focus of these chapters goes beyond what animal meats we can and cannot eat. The point God was making in these passages is that He doesn't want His people to consume anything that is harmful to their bodies. Jesus would not have put anything harmful in His body, which would have ensured He lived His life at His ideal body weight.

Now look again at Deuteronomy 14:2-3.

"For thou art an holy people unto the LORD thy God, and the LORD hath chosen thee to be a peculiar people unto himself, above all the nations that

are upon the earth. Thou shalt not eat any abominable thing." *(Deuteronomy 14:2-3, KJV).*

And also look again at I Corinthians 6:19-20.

"What? Know ye not that your body is the temple of the Holy Ghost which is in you, which ye have of God, and ye are not your own? For ye are bought with a price: therefore glorify God in your body, and in your spirit, which are God's." (I Corinthians 6:19-20, KJV)

Your light is to shine before men. You are to live above all nations. And you are to glorify God in your body. And God clearly communicates that a healthy diet, His diet, is essential to achieving those things in your life. These are things that God wants to accomplish in His people's lives today, just as He wanted to accomplish those things in His people's lives before Christ came.

How is it that anyone could read these three passages (Mark 5:16-19, Deut 14:2-3, and I Cor 6:19-20), along with Leviticus 11 and the remainder of Deuteronomy 14, and determine that God cared about our health and had a plan for our diets before Jesus came, but that Jesus' mission on Earth would result in a 'new truth' that would destroy these dietary laws, and that God no longer cares about our health and no longer has a plan for our diets? And how is it that we are supposed to glorify God in our bodies and have results far above all the nations if we don't honor what God is saying throughout these passages? We can't!!! That is why dietary deception in the Church is so important to Satan.

There was nothing that Jesus accomplished on the cross that changed God's concern for your health or the commandments He designed to ensure it. There is nothing that Jesus' work on the cross would have done to change the human body so that adherence to God's dietary directives was needed before Jesus came but was no longer necessary after Jesus came.

When the Church sees the word 'fulfill' it tries to argue that Jesus 'wrapped up' the need for the Old Testament commandments regarding diet. But that doesn't hold water. He goes on to say that those who obey and teach those commandments will be blessed. The only things that Jesus 'wrapped up' were the ceremonial and sacrificial practices designed to point to His coming and that gave God's people access to Him through the high priest.

Would we argue that the Ten Commandments no longer apply as well? The Church has got to quit picking and choosing what it wants to believe applies to us today from the Old Testament and what doesn't. Don't let anyone try to deceive you into believing that Deuteronomy 14 only applied to God's people at that time, another component of dietary deception that will keep you from your ideal body weight. Jesus would not have fallen prey to dietary deception; therefore, He would have lived His life at His ideal body weight.

Let's look once again at I Corinthians 6:19-20.

"What? Know ye not that your body is the temple of the Holy Ghost which is in you, which ye have of God, and ye are not your own? For ye are bought with a price: therefore glorify God in your body, and in your spirit, which are God's." (I Corinthians 6:19-20, KJV)

Nobody could have ever proven out their belief that their body was not their own and that they should glorify God in their body more than Jesus. He took that Biblical reality to the ultimate extent in His suffering and death on the cross. Someone who saw God as the owner of their body as much as Jesus did would have walked in obedience to God's dietary directives, ensuring that Jesus lived His life at His ideal body weight.

I emphasized earlier in the book that spiritual conditioning through Bible study, prayer, and worship was essential to successful living, certainly providing the necessary strength and self-control (fruit of the

Spirit) to walk in obedience to God's dietary directives. I think we would all contend that Jesus was the most spiritually conditioned person to ever walk this Earth, even to the point of obedience on the cross.

Based on His knowledge of Scripture, Jesus obviously meditated upon Scriptures extensively. And then we have numerous accounts of Jesus seeking His Father in times of prayer. And Jesus' entire life was an act of worship to His Father. You can be sure that Jesus would have been spiritually conditioned enough to walk in obedience to God's dietary directives, ensuring that He would have lived His live at His ideal body weight.

If Jesus had 'fallen off the wagon' and gained an excessive amount of weight (which He wouldn't have), would He have been sensitive to the Holy Spirit's direction in bringing Him to repentance and obedience to God's dietary directives? I think we can contend that Jesus was extensively sensitive to the direction of Father God in His life. It was only the will of the Father that Jesus sought to do. So yes, even if Jesus had spent a season out of His Father's will (which He didn't and wouldn't), Jesus would have been sensitive to His Father's leading and would have been able to again reach and maintain His ideal body weight.

Would Jesus have had a tendency towards unhealthy eating, or addictive behaviors in general, due to a lack of purpose in His life? Obviously, Jesus was very purpose-driven. No one has ever had a more important purpose for their lives, our salvation through faith. At a very early age, Jesus was always 'about His Father's business.' Jesus would have had no need to drown out the pain of a meaningless life; therefore, I would contend that Jesus lived His life at His ideal body weight.

We know that Jesus came that we might live life more abundantly. Living a life at 25, 50, 75, 100+ pounds overweight is not a more abundant life. Jesus came that our lives might be enriched in every area. Do you think that disobedience to dietary holiness and its effect on your health and body weight is the kind of enriched life Jesus wants for you? Jesus came to enrich you in all things, certainly to include your health and body weight. Jesus would not have overturned the applicability of dietary holiness. And Jesus certainly would not have overturned it in His own life. So we can be sure that Jesus would have lived His life at His ideal body weight.

"I thank my God always on your behalf for the grace of God which is given you by Jesus Christ; That in every thing ye are enriched by him, in all utterance, and in all knowledge." (I Corinthians 1:4-5, KJV)

Would Jesus have been motivated to eat healthy and maintain His ideal body weight as a witness to the world of the wisdom and power of God? Jesus' ultimate purpose was to provide you with a path to eternal salvation through faith in Him, and to equip you through the gift of the Holy Spirit to help you live a successful life, one that would glorify God. Jesus would have been highly motivated to demonstrate the wisdom and power of God to the world, maintaining a positive witness at all times. So Jesus would have lived His life at His ideal body weight.

Would Jesus have had a righteous motivation to live out His life at His ideal body weight? Jesus lived a sinless life. He was never guilty of lust or fornication. He was never guilty of seeking fame. He was never guilty of seeking anything to feed His flesh. So yes, Jesus' motivation to live out His life at His ideal body weight would have been a righteous one. Jesus would have lived His life at His ideal body weight.

In our modern world, try to picture Jesus walking around with a soda and a cinnamon roll. Focus on your first gut reaction to that. If you will be honest with yourself your view of Jesus, your respect for Jesus, would have dropped a bit. You would expect Jesus to be walking around with a bottled water and an apple, if anything.

Jesus would not have been found 'living unto himself' with soda and cinnamon roll in hand. One of His goals on the cross was to enable us to 'no longer live unto ourselves.' Eating a donut is living unto yourself.

Eating an apple is living unto God. Because Jesus lived His life unto God and others, we can be sure that He would have lived His life at His ideal body weight.

"And that he died for all, that they which live should not henceforth live unto themselves, but unto him which died for them, and rose again." (II Corinthians 5:15, KJV)

You might simply argue that Jesus would have weighed His ideal body weight because He walked everywhere. I would submit to you that Jesus didn't live out His life at His ideal body weight because He walked everywhere, but that He was able to walk everywhere because dietary holiness equipped Him with a body capable of doing so.

So, What Would Jesus Weigh? His ideal body weight. Follow His example. Remember WWJW every time you make a dietary choice.

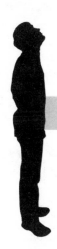
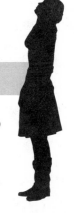

Chapter 22

Misinterpreted Scriptures That Keep You From Your Ideal Body Weight

In this chapter I have tried to cover every possible type of misconception and misinterpretation of Scripture of which I am aware that the Church has tried to use to overturn the Biblical principle of dietary holiness. I trust that you will find these sufficient to support the Biblical principle of dietary holiness demonstrated in this book.

In the event someone can point to a passage that 'seems' to contradict the applicability of dietary holiness to our lives, I would urge you to consider the preponderance of Biblical evidence available to you here, and to use the skills in Biblical dissection that this chapter, and this book, demonstrates. If anyone can read this book and still think they have found some 'loophole,' I would contend that this person does not have 'ears to hear' and is not open to the truth.

"… he that hath ears to hear, let him hear." (Luke 8:8, KJV)

"For every one that doeth evil hateth the light, neither cometh to the light, lest his deeds should be reproved." (John 3:20, KJV)

Gross Grace - Romans 14:1-21
Romans 14 is commonly known as the 'grace' chapter of the Bible. This passage is often used to argue that we are now free to do whatever we

want relative to diet because of what Jesus did on the cross. By now, I hope you realize how silly that is. Romans 14 deserves the distinction of being the 'most misinterpreted' chapter of the Bible.

The misinterpretation of Romans 14 is the way by which most fall victim to dietary deception. Let's thoroughly study this passage so we can do away with the stumbling block that has stood between God's people and the health He so desires for us through dietary holiness.

I realize that the following analysis may prove quite tedious. But please know that you are about to right the most common misinterpretation of Scripture in the Church, one that has kept you from your ideal body weight. Your patience and determination will pay off.

"1) *Receive one who is weak in the faith, but not to disputes over doubtful things.*

2) *For one believes he may eat all things, but he who is weak eats only vegetables.*

3) *Let not him who eats despise him who does not eat, and let not him who does not eat judge him who eats; for God has received him.*

4) *Who are you to judge another's servant? To his own master he stands or falls. Indeed, he will be made to stand, for God is able to make him stand.*

5) *One person esteems one day above another; another esteems every day alike. Let each be fully convinced in his own mind.*

6) *He who observes the day, observes it to the Lord; and he who does not observe the day, to the Lord he does not observe it. He who eats, eats to the Lord, for he gives God thanks; and he who does not eat, to the Lord he does not eat, and gives God thanks.*

7) *For none of us lives to himself, and no one dies to himself.*

8) *For if we live, we live to the Lord; and if we die, we die to the Lord. Therefore, whether we live or die, we are the Lord's.*

9) *For to this end Christ died and rose and lived again, that He might be Lord of both the dead and the living.*

10) *But why do you judge your brother? Or why do you show contempt for your brother? For we shall all stand before the judgment seat of Christ.*

11) *For it is written: "As I live, says the L*ORD*, Every knee shall bow to Me, And every tongue shall confess to God."*

12) *So then each of us shall give account of himself to God.*

13) *Therefore let us not judge one another anymore, but rather resolve this, not to put a stumbling block or a cause to fall in our brother's way.*

14) *I know and am convinced by the Lord Jesus that there is nothing unclean of itself; but to him who considers anything to be unclean, to him it is unclean.*

15) *Yet if your brother is grieved because of your food, you are no longer walking in love. Do not destroy with your food the one for whom Christ died.*

16) *Therefore do not let your good be spoken of as evil;*

17) *for the kingdom of God is not eating and drinking, but righteousness and peace and joy in the Holy Spirit.*

18) *For he who serves Christ in these things is acceptable to God and approved by men.*

19) *Therefore let us pursue the things which make for peace and the things by which one may edify another.*

20) *Do not destroy the work of God for the sake of food. All things indeed are pure, but it is evil for the man who eats with offense.*

21) *It is good neither to eat meat nor drink wine nor do anything by which your brother stumbles or is offended or is made weak." (Romans 14:1-21, NKJV, BibleGateway.com)*

Okay, let's carefully break this passage down. For starters, what is the context of the passage? The 'new Church' has just been formed through the one, final, perfect sacrifice of Jesus Christ. We now have salvation open to not only the Jews, but also to the Gentiles.

Over the centuries the Jews had developed their own man-made traditions and beliefs to honor God. And many of the Jews still held to the value of some of their former practices to honor God. The Gentiles, on the other hand, saw no value in esteeming one day over another in an effort to honor God, or in abstaining from certain foods on certain days in an effort to honor God, which were of the practices of the Jews. You can see the conflict coming already.

In Romans 14, Paul is trying to show the Believers how to react to, and view, one another regarding varied beliefs on how to best honor God. He is not trying to justify any type of sinful behavior, or any freedom regarding it. Paul is addressing matters that are open to opinion and individual conviction only.

A more modern example of this is that some in the Church believe that we should dress in a 3-piece suit or full-length dress on Sunday morning in order to properly honor God. While others see no reason why we shouldn't be able to wear a t-shirt, shorts, and flip-flops and honor God just as effectively through actions, words, and thoughts alone.

Now that we know the context, let's take on this passage one verse at a time.

Verse 1) Receive one who is weak in the faith, but not to disputes over doubtful things.

The Jews were 'weak in the faith' in that they felt they needed to adhere to their man-made beliefs regarding what would and would not be honoring to God. Their intentions were good. God is calling those who are not weak in faith to accept those who are, refusing to argue with those weak in faith over their beliefs and practices regarding how they choose to best honor God. Also, notice the term 'disputes over doubtful things.' The argument here is not about any clear law of Scripture such as 'do not eat pork.' The argument here is with regard to matters of opinion. There was no 'doubt' in anyone's mind, Jew and Gentile alike, that eating pork was a sin, for example.

Verse 2) For one believes he may eat all things, but he who is weak eats only vegetables.

On certain days, prior to the coming of Jesus Christ, the Jews might abstain from certain foods on certain days (animal meat for example). Some Jews still saw these practices as honoring to God.

The Gentiles saw no value in changing their diets from one day to the next. This is not a verse that justifies a sinful diet of junk non-foods, although the Church wants to interpret it that way, and has. The 'eat all things' text here is talking about foods designed and prescribed by God, not soda, donuts, cookies, and ham sandwiches. 'Eating all things' applies to God-approved foods only. It was only a question of whether or not to pull everything out of the diet except herbs on a particular day in order to honor God.

The issue was that the Jews determined that they should abstain from animal meats and eat only herbs on a particular day in order to honor God. The animal meats that applied were 'clean', not 'unclean'. No food eaten or not eaten was unhealthy. Unhealthy things like pork and donuts were not in the equation to begin with.

Verse 3) Let not him who eats despise him who does not eat, and let not him who does not eat judge him who eats; for God has received him.

The Gentiles were not to judge and despise those 'weak in faith' (the Jews) for abstaining from certain foods on certain days, nor were those 'weak in faith' (the Jews) to judge and despise the Gentiles who did not abstain. Pork and donuts were not in the equation, already understood to be off-limits by all, Jews and Gentiles alike.

Verse 4) Who are you to judge another's servant? To his own master he stands or falls. Indeed, he will be made to stand, for God is able to make him stand.
This is further support of the points made for Verse 3.

Verse 5) One person esteems one day above another; another esteems every day alike. Let each be fully convinced in his own mind.

The Apostle Paul is saying that if one person believes he is honoring God with a certain practice on a certain day, then that is fine. If another person sees no value in those practices towards honoring God, then that is fine too. Let each man proceed as he determines best. These 'practices' are not related to direct commandments of God; open to each individual's personal convictions.

Verse 6) He who observes the day, observes it to the Lord; and he who does not observe the day, to the Lord he does not observe it. He who eats, eats to the Lord, for he gives God thanks; and he who does not eat, to the Lord he does not eat, and gives God thanks.

The Apostle Paul is saying that whatever practice or tradition you participate in, the main issue is whether or not you are doing it as unto the Lord, to honor Him and thank Him for His love and blessings. It is not saying that as long as we give thanks we can eat something unhealthy. A meal of ham sandwiches, chocolate cake, and soda is not honoring to God, no matter how thankful we might be. And there is no such thing as eating unhealthy foods 'to the Lord,' such things being an abomination to God as we saw in Deuteronomy 14.

Verse 7) For none of us lives to himself, and no one dies to himself.

Verse 8) For if we live, we live to the Lord; and if we die, we die to the Lord. Therefore, whether we live or die, we are the Lord's.

Verse 9) For to this end Christ died and rose and lived again, that He might be Lord of both the dead and the living.

The main goal of our existence is to be pleasing and honoring to God. The way we choose to do that may be different from one person to the next. But that is between the individual and God. This is not to say that lying, stealing, and eating junk non-foods are okay for one person and not another. An unhealthy, gluttonous diet is sinful and wrong for all people, and does not constitute 'living to the Lord' but rather 'living to ourselves.'

Verse 10) But why do you judge your brother? Or why do you show contempt for your brother? For we shall all stand before the judgment seat of Christ.

Verse 11) For it is written: "As I live, says the LORD, *Every knee shall bow to Me, And every tongue shall confess to God."*

Verse 12) So then each of us shall give account of himself to God.

Verse 13) Therefore let us not judge one another anymore, but rather resolve this, not to put a stumbling block or a cause to fall in our brother's way.
Again, such differences in practices for pleasing and honoring God are between the individual and God. And it will be God who judges the intentions of the individual's heart, not other men. To argue that what someone else is doing is wrong is to create a stumbling block, or conflict, in their minds as to what they believe they should or shouldn't do to honor God. The 'practices' in question would not include lying, stealing, and eating pork, for example, but things, in and of themselves, that are not sinful; matters of opinion.

Verse 14) I know and am convinced by the Lord Jesus that there is nothing unclean of itself; but to him who considers anything to be unclean, to him it is unclean.
The Apostle Paul is talking about the difference in practices. He is not saying Twinkies are clean, or okay. He is, again, talking about those practices or traditions, which in and of themselves, do not constitute sin and in no way violate Godly principles. Twinkies, a destructive substance to spirit, soul, and body, do violate God's principles, character,

and desire for His people. But if you believe wearing anything other than a suit or dress to church is wrong, then for you to not wear a suit or dress to church is unclean for you, although not necessarily unclean for others.

Verse 15) Yet if your brother is grieved because of your food, you are no longer walking in love. Do not destroy with your food the one for whom Christ died.

Verse 16) Therefore do not let your good be spoken of as evil;
Even though your practices may not constitute sin, if they offend your brother, then you are to abstain from them for their sake. There is no reason for your 'good', what you believe to be the best way to honor God, to receive the judgment of others. But anyone who walked into the congregation with a ham sandwich and soda would have offended all, these not being neutral practices, but sinful practices.

Verse 17) for the kingdom of God is not eating and drinking, but righteousness and peace and joy in the Holy Spirit.
The Apostle Paul is not 'okaying' junk non-foods and unclean animal meats. He is saying that whether you eat or don't eat certain foods, God-approved foods, <u>on certain days</u>, the kingdom of God is about more important things than such man-made traditions.

Verse 18) For he who serves Christ in these things is acceptable to God and approved by men.
If our heart's intent is to please God through our man-made traditions, then God finds them acceptable, and they should not receive the condemnation of man.

Verse 19) Therefore let us pursue the things which make for peace and the things by which one may edify another.

So do not argue over tradition and differences in the way we choose to honor God, but rather focus on those things that edify one another. By the way, walking in obedience to dietary holiness, and teaching others to do the same, edifies other Believers.

Verse 20) Do not destroy the work of God for the sake of food. All things indeed are pure, but it is evil for the man who eats with offense.
'All things' applies to clean animal meats and herbs, for example, not unclean animal meats and donuts. God's foods will not destroy the work of God, regardless of our man-made traditions. However, we know that junk non-foods do in fact destroy the work of God as they serve to destroy us in spirit, soul, and body.

Verse 21) It is good neither to eat meat nor drink wine nor do anything by which your brother stumbles or is offended or is made weak.
Here is the whole conclusion of the matter, the entire purpose for Romans 14. We are not to create stumbling blocks for other Believers by insisting that their traditions are wrong, and that our traditions are right. This does not apply to things that are explicitly sinful like lying, stealing, and unhealthy eating.

Each is to make up his own mind in regard to what practices he wants to use to honor God, and not be confused or diverted by the beliefs of others and their man-made traditions and practices to honor God. Nor are we to create a stumbling block by eating certain foods in front of them on days they believe we should abstain. And again, as I have made so perfectly clear, it is talking about God's food, not unhealthy non-foods, the destructive qualities of which affect all persons.

I realize that was a bit long and tedious, but it is worth grinding through Romans 14 to get to the bottom of one of the sources of dietary deception, to understand what Romans 14 is really saying.

Dirty Deeds - Mark 7

Mark 7 is another passage used to support dietary deception, the belief that God's dietary directives no longer apply to us because of the work of Christ on the cross. Mark 7 is one of the most grossly misinterpreted passages of the Bible, even modified, in the Church's willful attempt to justify the desires of its sinful flesh.

Mark 7 is a commonly misinterpreted passage. We have taken it from 'Jesus said that some dirt on the food (God's food) will not harm us spiritually and physically' to 'Jesus said we can eat anything we want.' How convenient. With that kind of Biblical study and interpretation, and the willing denial of the truth to satisfy the desires of our flesh, is it any wonder the Church has become so tired, sick, and overweight?

Let me start with the conclusion and then prove it out. The point of this passage was that we need to 'wash our hearts from evil' (God's commandment), and not be so concerned about 'keeping the dirt off our food' (man's tradition).

Having covered Romans 14, Mark 7 will be much more easily understood, as we have learned to take Scripture in context and to discern its meaning and application. Let's now look at Mark 7:1-23 and do the same as we consider the dialogue between Jesus and the Pharisees and scribes.

"1) *Then came together unto him the Pharisees, and certain of the scribes, which came from Jerusalem.*

2) *And when they saw some of his disciples eat bread with defiled, that is to say, with unwashen hands, they found fault.*

3) *For the Pharisees, and all the Jews, except they wash their hands oft, eat not, holding the tradition of the elders.*

4) *And when they come from the market, except they wash, they eat not, and many other things there be, which they have received to hold, as the washing of cups, and pots, brazen vessels, and of tables.*

5) *Then the Pharisees and scribes asked him, why walk not thy disciples*

according to the tradition of the elders, but eat bread with unwashen hands?

6) *He answered and said unto them, Well hath Esaias prophesied of you hypocrites, as it is written, This people honoureth me with their lips, but their heart is far from me.*

7) *Howbeit in vain do they worship me, teaching for doctrines the commandments of men.*

8) *For laying aside the commandment of God, ye hold the tradition of men, as the washing of pots and cups: and many other such like things ye do.*

9) *And he said unto them, Full well ye reject the commandment of God, that ye may keep your own tradition.*

10) *For Moses said, Honour thy father and thy mother; and, Whoso curseth father or mother, let him die the death:*

11) *But ye say, If a man shall say to his father or mother, It is Corban, that is to say, a gift, by whatsoever thou mightest be profited by me; he shall be free.*

12) *And ye suffer him no more to do ought for his father or mother;*

13) *Making the word of God of none effect through your tradition, which ye have delivered: and many such like things do ye.*

14) *And when he had called all the people unto him, he said unto them, Hearken unto me every one of you, and understand:*

15) *There is nothing from without a man, that entering into him can defile him: but the things which come out of him, those are they that defile the man.*

16) *If any man have ears to hear, let him hear.*

17) *And when He was entered into the house from the people, His disciples asked Him concerning the parable.*

18) *And He saith unto them, Are ye so without understanding also? Do ye not perceive, that whatever thing from without entereth into the man, it cannot defile him.*

19) *Because it entereth not into his heart, but into the belly, and goeth out into the draught, purging all meats?*

20) *And he said, That which cometh out of the man, that defileth the man.*

21) *For from within, out of the heart of men, proceed evil thoughts, adulteries, fornications, murders,*

22) *Thefts, covetousness, wickedness, deceit, lasciviousness, an evil eye, blasphemy, pride, foolishness:*

23) *All these evil things come from within, and defile the man."* (Mark 7:1-23, KJV)

The point of the passage is that we need to 'wash our hearts from evil' (God's commandment), and not be so concerned about 'keeping the dirt off our food' (man's tradition). It is the heart that counts, not some man-made tradition. The Pharisees followed man-made traditions and judged others who didn't, but they did not have hearts that were right towards God. The disciples did not follow man-made traditions, and they did have hearts that were right towards God.

We know that this passage is not referring to unclean meats because the Pharisees were focused on the dirt that might get on the food and nothing else. Believe me, if the food involved in this account had been pork, the Pharisees would have been so upset about that in this account that the mention of dirty hands would have never even been made. Actually, the food involved wasn't animal meat at all, it was bread. Keep in mind that this would have been healthy bread. Man's perverted refinement processes had not yet been devised at this point in history.

In no way whatsoever is this passage indicating that Jesus said it is okay to have a ham sandwich, coke, and candy bar for lunch. These are unclean non-foods. The 'meats' referred to in Mark 7:19 would have not included unclean animal meats or donuts. For this passage, the actual food eaten was bread, which leads me to believe that 'meats' in this case is a general application to all types of God-approved foods.

Only God's prescribed and designated foods are clean, whether they have some dirt on them or not. Satan's perverted non-foods are 'not clean' or not healthy for the body, whether or not they have some dirt on them. A 'spotless' donut is still 'not clean.'

Now let's look at the most disturbing component of the Biblical misinterpretation surrounding Mark 7, specifically Mark 7:19. In numerous Biblical translations, the literal and intentional modification of Scripture by man has been made to ensure the justified fulfillment of man's flesh in the area of diet. This is a major issue that needs to be addressed in a formal manner by the 'Biblical authorities,' whoever they may be.

Let's consider two Biblical translations of Mark 7:19 to illustrate my strong claim, the King James Version (correct) and the New International Version (incorrect). There are actually worse translations than the NIV out there in this regard.

"Because it entereth not into his heart, but into the belly, and goeth out into the draught, purging all meats?" (Mark 7:19, KJV)

"For it doesn't go into their heart but into their stomach, and then out of the body. (In saying this, Jesus declared all foods clean.)" (Mark 7:19, NIV, BibleGateway.com)

The King James Version tells us that the dirt on the food doesn't affect, enter into, a man's heart. It tells us that the dirt on the food will go into the stomach and be filtered out, or purged, by our digestive systems. In no way is this verse referring to 'unclean meats'. It is emphasizing the dirt on approved, clean foods. And that is all. The emphasis is on the dirt, not the food.

The New International Version also tells us that the dirt on the food doesn't affect, enter into, a man's heart. It tells us that the dirt on the food will be handled by our stomachs and digestive systems as well. So far, so good.

But then we come to a man-made addition, a man-made interpretation actually, that tells us that Mark 7 is saying that 'Jesus has declared all foods clean.' Notice how they carefully used the term 'clean' in an effort to overcome any possibility of the Church ever walking in dietary holiness, or being required to do so. Nothing could be more misleading. If the NIV Bible wants to include its own interpretations along the way then maybe its name should be changed to the NIV Commentary.

Relative to diet, what 'Jesus declared' was that 'the dirt on the food you eat will be filtered out by your digestive system' and that 'the dirt on food will not enter your heart.' Nothing more and nothing less. It is Biblical heresy for those responsible for the NIV and other translations to leave this addition in 'their' versions of the Bible. Go to 'biblos.com' and do your own review of the Greek text to see that such verbiage does not, or should not, exist.

In no way was Jesus communicating that you are now free to eat any unclean thing you want. That is ludicrous. Like I said before, gluttony and junk non-foods are the Church's drug of choice, its secret sin. And the Church will misinterpret, and even modify, Scripture to justify this secret sin and to cover up this fleshly conspiracy.

Somebody (not Jesus) thought it necessary to 'help us along' with an addition to the NIV version of the verse, at least highlighted by the fact that this addition is in parenthesis in the NIV. Some versions don't even put this addition in parenthesis. The Church acts like this addition, this man-made interpretation, is part of Scripture. It isn't. It clearly sticks out like a sore thumb as something that doesn't belong there, and isn't an accurate interpretation atop that. This misinterpretation and man-made addition to Mark 7:19 is one of the leading causes of dietary deception that has kept the Church from dietary holiness, the very reason the Church is tired, sick, and overweight.

Freedom Foolishness – Romans 6:1-2

God's grace, His gift of salvation through faith and faith alone, despite our sinfulness, was not meant to provide us with a license to continue in sin. Or in the case of dietary holiness, which the Church has worked hard to deny even exists, God's grace was never meant to free us from His dietary directives, His standard for holy living in the area of diet.

If you are reading this book you know that a license to sin in the area of diet has resulted in anything but freedom. It has resulted in enslavement and suffering. Freedom is not life without standards for holy living. Freedom, if anything, as a Believer, is being equipped through Bible study, prayer, worship, and the indwelling of the Holy Spirit to walk in victory in every area of your life, health and body weight most certainly included.

Victory in the area of health, in reaching and maintaining your ideal body weight, requires adherence to God's dietary directives. Period! End of discussion. Jesus' work on the cross would have never been intended to take away the very path you must travel to reach your ideal body weight and good health. Do you see the insanity of it all?

We are not living in freedom when we find ourselves unable, or unwilling, to control the behaviors in our lives that work to harm us. I can do without that kind of freedom. That is freedom foolishness.

"What shall we say then? Shall we continue in sin that grace may abound? God forbid. How shall we, that are dead in sin, live any longer therein?" (Romans 6:1-2, KJV)

Do we really think that God purchased the right to have ownership of our bodies through the life, death, and resurrection of Jesus Christ only to hand it back over to us to destroy?

"What! Know ye not that your body is the temple of the Holy Spirit which is in you, which ye have of God, and ye are not your own?" (I Corinthians 6:19, KJV)

"I beseech you therefore, brethren, by the mercies of God, that ye present your bodies a living sacrifice, holy, acceptable unto God, which is your reasonable

service. And be not conformed to the pattern of this world, but be you transformed by the renewing of your mind, that you may prove what is that good, acceptable, and perfect will of God." (Romans 12:1-2, KJV)

An overweight body is not acceptable to God, or the path to it. This is not the good, acceptable, and perfect will of God for you. This is not God's will for your life. Living your life at your ideal body weight is your birthright as a Believer.

Fulfillment Fallacy – Matthew 5:16-19

Parts of this section will be the duplication of an explanation regarding this passage that I made earlier, but I think it is worth repeating.

"Let your light so shine before men, that they may see your good works, and glorify your Father which is in Heaven. Think not that I am come to destroy the law, or the prophets: I am not come to destroy, but to fulfill. For verily I say unto you, till heaven and earth pass, one jot or one tittle shall in no wise pass from the law, till all be fulfilled. Whosoever therefore shall break one of these least commandments, and shall teach men so, he shall be called the least in the kingdom of heaven: but whosoever shall do and teach them, the same shall be called great in the kingdom of heaven." (Matthew 5:16-19, KJV)

These are the words of Jesus Himself. How is it that the Church has been able to convince itself that the dietary directives of God no longer apply to us today after reading a passage like this? Through dietary deception, which involves our fleshly desires, we have been enticed to misinterpret, even modify, Scripture to support our ways.

Jesus' purpose on this Earth was not to destroy the law. And I think it is safe for us to assume He was fully aware of Leviticus 11 and Deuteronomy 14 when He said that. As you may recall, in these chapters God spelled out what animal meats should (clean) and should not (unclean) be eaten. The main focus of these chapters goes beyond what animal meats we can and cannot eat. The point God was making in these passages is that He doesn't want His people to consume anything that is harmful to their bodies.

Now look again at Deuteronomy 14:2-3.

"For thou art an holy people unto the LORD thy God, and the LORD hath chosen thee to be a peculiar people unto himself, above all the nations that are upon the earth. Thou shalt not eat any abominable thing." (Deuteronomy 14:2-3, KJV).

And also look again at I Corinthians 6:19-20.

"What? Know ye not that your body is the temple of the Holy Ghost which is in you, which ye have of God, and ye are not your own? For ye are bought with a price: therefore glorify God in your body, and in your spirit, which are God's." (I Corinthians 6:19-20, KJV)

Your light is to shine before men. You are to live above all nations. And you are to glorify God in your body. And God clearly communicates that a healthy diet, His diet, is essential to achieving those things in your life. These are things that God wants to accomplish in His people's lives today, just as He wanted to accomplish those things in His people's lives before Christ came.

How is it that anyone could read these three passages (Mark 5:16-19, Deut 14:2-3, and I Cor 6:19-20), along with Leviticus 11 and the remainder of Deuteronomy 14, and determine that God cared about our health and had a plan for our diets before Jesus came, but that Jesus' mission on Earth would result in a 'new truth' that would destroy these dietary laws, and that God no longer cares about our health and no longer has a plan for our diets? And how is it that we are supposed to glorify God in our bodies and have results far above all the nations if we don't honor what God is saying throughout these passages? We can't!!! That is why dietary deception in the Church is so important to Satan.

There was nothing that Jesus accomplished on the cross that changed God's concern for your health or the commandments He designed to ensure it. There is nothing that Jesus' work on the cross would have done to change the human body so that adherence to God's dietary directives was needed before Jesus came but was no longer necessary after Jesus came.

When the Church sees the word 'fulfill' it tries to argue that Jesus 'wrapped up' the need for the Old Testament commandments regarding diet. But that doesn't hold water. He goes on to say that those who obey and teach those commandments will be blessed. The only things that Jesus 'wrapped up' were the ceremonial and sacrificial practices designed to point to His coming and that gave God's people access to Him through the high priest.

Would we argue that the Ten Commandments no longer apply as well? The Church has got to quit picking and choosing what it wants to believe applies to us today from the Old Testament and what doesn't. Don't let anyone try to deceive you into believing that Deuteronomy 14 only applied to God's people at that time; another component of dietary deception that will keep you from your ideal body weight.

Let me give you a striking example that supports that the dietary and cleanliness laws of the Old Testament still apply to us today. Before getting to the example you must first consider Numbers 19:11, which addresses a cleanliness law concerning the handling of dead human bodies.

"He that toucheth the dead body of any man shall be unclean seven days." (Numbers 19:11, KJV)

In the mid-1800's, before the development of the 'germ theory of disease,' lived a Hungarian physician by the name of Ignaz Semmelweis. By the way, God already addressed the 'germ theory of disease' in His cleanliness laws several thousands of years before that. He just chose not to get all 'scientific' on us. It is ours to obey, not always to understand. Strangely enough, it is often through our desire to understand that we get so off course. We tend to think we can out-smart God and come up with our own philosophies of how we should live our lives. Here is a perfect example, with devastating consequences.

Dr. Semmelweis worked in a clinic that practiced the examination of pregnant women. This clinic also examined dead bodies. The average death rate for the women involved in these examinations was a horrible 10%, even as high as 18.3% in April, 1847. Dr. Semmelweis was beside himself with concern, as of course he should have been.

The common practice of the medical students in his clinic was to examine dead bodies to start the day and then move on to the examination of the pregnant women. Dr. Semmelweis theorized that the medical students might be carrying contaminants of some sort from the dead bodies to the pregnant women. He began to insist that the medical students thoroughly wash their hands after examining the dead bodies. In a three month period, the monthly death rate for the pregnant women dropped from 18.3% to below 2%, even to zero in some months.

Did Dr. Semmelweis win the respect of the medical community? Did he win a Nobel Peace Prize? No. He was mocked, slandered, and ran out of his practice for daring to highlight a failure in the medical community, despite statistics that were remarkable and uncontestable as valid and true.

This is the same spirit of deception that is working today in opposition to dietary holiness. I fully expect this book to excite a similar attack on me from many in the Church. But I must answer God's call on my life in this regard and teach the truth of dietary holiness just the same. I am happy to report that Dr. Semmelweis is now considered a pioneer of antiseptic procedures.

After reading about this story, can you argue that the Jesus' work on the cross did away with all the cleanliness laws and our responsibility to obey them today? Can you argue that touching a dead human's body would not make you a serious health threat to yourself and to others? No way. Then you can't argue that the dietary laws no longer apply to us today either. You will know evil by its evil fruit.

"A good tree cannot bring forth evil fruit; neither can a corrupt tree bring forth good fruit... by their fruits ye shall know them." (Matthew 7:18-20, KJV)

"For a good tree bringeth not forth corrupt fruit, neither doth a corrupt tree bring forth good fruit, for every tree is known by his own fruit..." (Luke 6:43-44, KJV)

The reason Jesus came was to provide a way for each of us to have a personal relationship with God and to give us the indwelling of the Holy Spirit. No longer are we required to offer sacrifices for our sins. Jesus was the ultimate and final sacrifice. No longer are we required to have access to God only through the priests and the prophets. We can each approach God personally. No longer are the ceremonial laws needed to point ahead to Jesus' coming. He already came. But Jesus did not come to do away with the dietary and cleanliness laws designed to bless and protect us. We have been foolish to argue otherwise.

If you want to argue that God's Old Testament dietary directives no longer apply to you today, then you will have a hard time praying Psalm 119:18.

"Open thou mine eyes, that I may behold wondrous things out of thy law." (Psalm 119:18, KJV)

If you are not open to the truth and value of God's dietary directives then you will not experience the 'wondrous things' from God's law that

He designed to bless you and to make your life a witness to the world, a light on a hill, and one above all the nations.

And relative to the 'liberty' we argue we have in Christ to do whatever we want in the area of diet and health, God tells us that obeying His law is where liberty (freedom from enslavement and destruction) can be found.

"So shall I keep thy law continually for ever and ever. And I will walk at liberty: for I seek thy precepts." (Psalm 119:44-45, KJV)

'For ever and ever' would surely include today. Jesus' sacrifice on the cross was not intended to deliver us from the very Biblical precepts that provide us with true liberty and blessing. Our enslavement to unhealthy eating, and its destructive impact, is an example of a loss of liberty in the Church, not a supposed freedom to be enjoyed.

Moderation Madness – Philippians 4:5

Almost no matter what the subject, certainly to include diet, we will often justify our deviations from the best choices (and God's commands) for our lives by stating 'all things in moderation.' It appears that most people believe this to be a Biblical principle. This is a tragic misinterpretation and misapplication of Philippians 4:5.

"Let your moderation be known unto all men." (Philippians 4:5, KJV)

There is a big difference between 'all things in moderation', the common take-away, and 'showing moderation to all men,' what it actually says. God would not be telling us to moderate our adultery or to moderate our stealing, nor is He saying that we should moderately eat unhealthy things. God requires abstinence from sin, not moderation of it.

God is talking about demonstrating a control over those things that are not in and of themselves harmful. For example, in and of itself, golf is not harmful. However, if we become obsessed with it and begin playing so often that our relationship with God and our family suffers, we have not been obedient to Philippians 4:5. Titus 2:11-12 helps to lend to this topic.

"For the grace of God that bringeth salvation hath appeared to all men, teaching us that, denying ungodliness and worldly lusts, we should live soberly, righteously, and godly, in this present world." (Titus 2:11-12, KJV)

You don't control evil. Evil controls you. You are not to toy with evil. You are to flee from evil. You will find that abstaining from refined sugars, for example, is much easier than trying to moderate them.

I realize this is contrary to Weight Watchers' latest slogan, 'You can have your cake and lose weight too. Eat real food in the real world.' This is man's way, not God's Weigh. This is not the wisdom and path that will sustain you long-term. Don't allow sinful behaviors, no matter how seemingly small, to maintain a foothold in your life.

You may very well find, as I did, that is easier to make one decision to avoid cookies, for example, all together, than to have to make multiple decisions about whether to have any, and if so, how many, and then exercising volume control, etc. Total abstinence from sin is easier than trying to moderate and control sin.

"… make not provision for the flesh, to fulfill the lusts thereof." (Romans 13:14, KJV)

Avoiding moderation madness will help to ensure that you reach and maintain your ideal body weight.

Permissive Perversion – I Corinthians 10:23
All things are permissible under the new covenant, right? That is certainly what the Church wants to believe. We even think that is what the Bible says, somewhere.

"All things are lawful for me, but all things are not expedient: all things are lawful for me, but all things edify not." (I Corinthians 10:23, KJV)

To begin with, would we argue that 'all things' includes stealing, adultery, or dishonoring our parents? Of course not, yet we argue that 'all things' includes destroying our bodies through sinful dietary practices.

I think the 'all things are not expedient (or beneficial)' is the real tricky part; that is, if we fail to study this verse within its context. We might, and have, concluded that even though our dietary practices may not be beneficial to our bodies, this verse gives us the divine 'okay' to do so anyway.

And what about the 'but all things edify not.' 'But' is an important twist in this verse. Whatever it is that we are 'allowed' to do, it is saying that 'it may not edify' others. Or in other words, if the activity talked about here is not helpful, encouraging, and beneficial to others, we should abstain from it.

Okay, but what is the 'activity' that is being discussed here? Is it talking about something specific, or does it apply to 'all things,' to include our dietary practices? Let's look to this passage in its full context so we can know what God is talking about here.

"18) Behold Israel after the flesh: are not they which eat of the sacrifices partakers of the altar?

19) What say I then? That the idol is any thing, or that which is offered in sacrifice to idols is any thing?

20) But I say, that the things which the Gentiles sacrifice, they sacrifice to devils, and not to God: and I would not that ye should have fellowship with devils.

21) Ye cannot drink the cup of the Lord, and the cup of devils: ye cannot be partakers of the Lord's table, and of the table of devils.

22) Do we provoke the Lord to jealousy? Are we stronger than He?

23) *All things are lawful for me, but all things are not expedient: all things are lawful for me, but all things edify not.*

24) *Let no man see his own, but every man another's wealth.*

25) *Whatever is sold in the shamble, that eat, asking no question for conscience sake:*

26) *For the earth is the Lord's, and the fullness thereof.*

27) *If any of them that believe not, and ye be disposed to go; whatsoever is set before you, eat, asking no question for conscience sake that showed it, and for conscience sake: for the earth is the Lord's, and the fullness thereof.*

29) *Conscience, I say, not thine own, but of the other: for why is my liberty judged of another man's conscience?*

30) *For if I by grace be a partaker, why am I evil spoken of for that for which I give thanks?*

31) *Whether therefore ye eat, or drink, or whatsover ye do, do all to the glory of God."* (I Corinthians 10:1-31, KJV)

To summarize, thereby clarifying the common misinterpretation of Scripture relative to I Corinthians 10:23, let's carefully work through this passage.

Verse 18) Behold Israel after the flesh: are not they which eat of the sacrifices partakers of the altar?
The Apostle Paul is talking about eating foods formally sacrificed to idols. The question is an effort to determine whether or not it is okay for God's people to eat something formally sacrificed to idols. Evidently, for some, to do so seemed wrong. For them, to see someone willingly eat of meat formally sacrificed to idols, in their conscience, meant that person was someone who has in effect partaken in idol worship themselves, by association if nothing else.

Then there were others who saw no concern with eating foods formally sacrificed to idols. They saw that the food was good for nourishment and felt no association with the idol worship that may have occurred before. They did not feel like the consumption of that food made them partakers with anything evil.

The issue here does not involve any unclean animal meats or substances of which God did not approve. The substances considered here are only God-approved foods. The food type itself was not the issue addressed here. Had the sacrificed flesh been roast pork, it would have been understood by all that this was unclean to eat, whether or not formally part of idol worship.

Verse 19) What say I then? That the idol is any thing, or that which is offered in sacrifice to idols is any thing?
The Apostle Paul indicated that the value of the sacrificed meat relative to nourishment is not affected by any sacrificial ceremony. The evil ceremonial practices of non-believers are of no practical, physical consequence for the Believer in this regard. There is nothing that idol worship could have done that would have given Satan any power to corrupt God's created foods.

Verse 20) But I say, that the things which the Gentiles sacrifice, they sacrifice to devils, and not to God: and I would not that ye should have fellowship with devils.
The Apostle Paul assures everyone where he is coming from, that he certainly would not want anyone to have fellowship with devils. He is not trying to justify any such worship as acceptable; however, he works to point out that this is not what is being performed by those who simply want the meat for food.

Verses 21 & 22) Ye cannot drink the cup of the Lord, and the cup of devils: ye cannot be partakers of the Lord's table, and of the table of devils. Do we provoke the Lord to jealousy? Are we stronger than He?

If we truly worship the Lord God of Heaven, simply eating the meat formally sacrificed to idols will not then make us a part of those who worship Satan.

Verses 23 & 24) All things are lawful for me, but all things are not expedient: all things are lawful for me, but all things edify not. Let no man see his own, but every man another's wealth.

Although it may be of no consequence to one person to eat of the meat formally sacrificed to idols, it may be non-edifying to someone else who is weaker in faith or with a sensitive conscience in that regard. Therefore, the proper response by the one who has no concerns over the consumption of the sacrificed meat is to consider the other person's welfare, and abstain.

Verse 25) Whatever is sold in the shamble, that eat, asking no question for conscience sake:

The Apostle Paul further clarifies that the effect of the sacrificed meat on one's body is of no consequence. He encourages us to not even inquire as to whether or not the meat has been sacrificed to idols or not, thereby ensuring that it does not hinder our faith, or someone else's faith, in any way.

Verses 26 through 31) For the earth is the Lord's, and the fullness thereof. If any of them that believe not, and ye be disposed to go; whatsoever is set before you, eat, asking no question for conscience sake that showed it, and for conscience sake: for the earth is the Lord's, and the fullness thereof. Conscience, I say, not thine own, but of the other: for why is my liberty judged of another man's conscience? For if I by grace be a partaker, why am I evil spoken of for that for which I give thanks? Whether therefore ye eat, or drink, or whatsover ye do, do all to the glory of God.

The Apostle Paul goes on to further support the messages of verses 18 to 25 by 1) emphasizing that all of creation is from God. (i.e. no ceremonial practices of man, even something as evil as sacrificing meat to idols, has any power over God's created foods), 2) encouraging us to act in such a way so as to be of greatest benefit to our fellow man, 3) asking us to resist the tendency to judge another's weaker conscience and for others to resist the tendency to judge our sense of greater liberty, and 4) showing us that it is the condition of the individual's heart that matters, not whether or not the meat had been formerly sacrificed to idols.

And relative to 'do all to the glory of God,' no one who is partaking in an unhealthy diet is 'doing so to the glory of God.' As noted before, an unhealthy and overweight body is not glorifying to God.

I believe I have made it clear that this passage has nothing whatsoever to do with God's attempt to 'okay' eating body-destroying, perversions of His created foods. Had the sacrificed meat instead been soda, candy, and pork, then there would have in fact been an issue with its consumption, whether sacrificed to idols or not.

Dining Deception – Luke 10:8 & I Corinthians 10:27
Many would argue that the right thing to do when you sit down at someone's table is to eat what is offered you, no matter what it might be. They would argue that such a belief came from the Bible. The Bible says 'eat whatever is set before you,' right? Let's more carefully consider that common misconception and Scriptural misinterpretation.

"And into whatsoever city ye enter, and they receive you, eat such things as are set before you:" (Luke 10:8, KJV)

This is not an example of Jesus approving the consumption of unclean animal meats and unclean anything. Jesus would no more ask His disciples to partake in eating unclean things in order to make their host feel more comfortable than He would ask His disciples to get drunk in order to make their alcoholic host feel more comfortable. This doesn't mean they will be partaking in the roast pork if offered.

The point here is that Jesus' disciples have earned the right to be fed and need not feel guilty about such a gift. Therefore, the disciples should freely accept the offer of food set before them. See the previous verse.

"And in the same house remain, eating and drinking such things as they give: for the labourer is worthy of his hire..." (Luke 10:7, KJV)

Although you may in fact offend the host by refusing to eat anything unhealthy that they might serve, that is none of your concern. Your concern is to put God first and walk in obedience to His Word. And besides, whether the host is offended or not, you will provide a witness of obedience to the host that they will never forget.

Another opportunity for confusion in this regard can be found in I Corinthians 10:27.

"... whatever is set before you, eat, asking no question for conscience sake." (I Corinthians 10:27, KJV)

As we covered earlier, I Corinthians 10 addresses the consumption of food formally sacrificed to idols. As you saw, the food involved would have been an approved food, no unclean animal meat or anything unhealthy at all. That was not the focus of this passage. The issue was that some were offended by others' consumption of foods formally sacrificed to idols, while others, recognizing that there was nothing that man or Satan could do to the food to change its value for nourishment, didn't have a problem with it.

The point of I Corinthians 10:27 specifically was that it is better not to ask if the food was formally sacrificed to idols, or to tell someone that it was formally sacrificed to idols. Knowing would simply create an issue for some, not an issue for others, and a conflict between the two sides.

Thanks Theory – Romans 14:6
Well, even if the meal served is unhealthy, as long as we give God thanks we are okay, right? Wrong. No amount of thanks in the world will change a breakfast of coffee and donuts into something nutritious for your body. This confusion may come from a misunderstanding of Romans 14:6

"… He who eats, eats to the Lord, for he gives God thanks; and he who does not eat, to the Lord he does not eat, and gives God thanks." (Romans 14:6, NKJV, BibleGateway.com)

As we saw earlier, the Apostle Paul is saying that whatever practice or tradition you participate in, the main issue is whether or not you are doing it as unto the Lord, to honor Him and thank Him for His love and blessings. It is not saying that as long as we give thanks we can eat something unhealthy. A meal of ham sandwiches, chocolate cake, and soda is not honoring to God, no matter how thankful we might be. And there is no such thing as eating unhealthy foods 'to the Lord', such things being an abomination to God as we saw in Deuteronomy 14.

It is utterly insane that we would ask God to bless the consumption of junk non-foods to the nourishment of our bodies. But it happens at almost any meal where a prayer is spoken. It doesn't seem to matter that the meal is made up of ham sandwiches, chocolate cake, and soda.

Giving thanks to God for your successful theft or your ongoing adulterous relationship will not miraculously change those sins into righteousness. Giving thanks to God for the unhealthy meal you are about to eat doesn't suddenly make it okay.

The stuff you are about to put into your mouth is either of God, and nutritious, or not of God, and poisonous. All the prayer in the world will not motivate God to change the chemical makeup of what you are about to eat. If it is a God-approved food, it will bless/nourish your body. If it is not a God-approved, it will curse/destroy your body.

Don't pray for health. Obey for health.

Shame Sham

Go to the chapter 'The Holy Spirit Leading You to Your Ideal Body weight' where shame, and its purpose in our lives, is discussed in detail. In this chapter we saw that to explain away the shame we might feel about being overweight as simply an issue of self-esteem or poor body image is a 'sham'. The shame we feel for being overweight is the working of the Holy Spirit in our lives to direct us back to God and His ways.

Conviction Copout

We so often hear from those who do not want to change their ways 'God hasn't convicted me of that.' Much like legalism, most Believers cannot practically define the term 'conviction,' much less make effective application.

What is conviction? Conviction is basically a strong belief. For the Christian, the definition of conviction becomes more precise, and can come in two basic forms. One form of conviction might be termed 'Biblical conviction,' which is simply the affect that God's explicit Biblical messages have on us. We see the truth that God has laid out in His Word for us, and because of the Holy Spirit that indwells in us, we believe it to be true, and hopefully we also act upon that belief. The topic of God's diet is more along these lines.

The second form is not based on a Biblical principle or directive. The second form might be termed 'circumstantial conviction.' In this form, the Holy Spirit works in us to lead us to a specific action and decision, one not explicitly addressed in Scripture.

For example, a pastor was recently given several hundred dollars for some ministry work he had performed at another church. He laid the money aside in an envelope on his desk, not really knowing what he should do with it. Over the course of the next week, every time the pastor looked at the envelope, a particular person's face was impressed upon his mind. Ultimately, the pastor felt 'convicted' that he should give the money to that person.

This second form does not apply to dietary holiness. The message of God's Word relative to diet is not variable or circumstantial. It was true yesterday, it is true today, and it will be true tomorrow, for all people.

Bogus Binding – I Corinthians 8:12-14

This is one of the more absurd misconceptions I have ever run across. The Bogus Binding of the Conscience philosophy is one that seems to basically argue that we don't want to offend anyone with a truth God has not made evident to them already, because to do so would be to put a burden upon them that didn't exist before (i.e. bind their conscience). That is an outrageous misinterpretation of Scripture that may have come from passages like I Corinthians 8:12-14.

"But when ye sin so against the brethren, and would wound their weak conscience, ye sin against Christ. Wherefore, if meat make my brother to offend, I will eat no flesh while the world standeth, lest I make my brother to offend." (I Corinthians 8:12-14, KJV)

This passage is talking about how to handle differences in beliefs as to whether or not it is okay to consume meats formally sacrificed to idols. We addressed that topic earlier with our study of I Corinthians 10. Those who are not okay with it have a 'weak conscience.' The point is that we should not eat meat formally sacrificed to idols, if others, of a 'weaker conscience,' are offended. This passage is not saying we should avoid presenting someone with a truth of God's Word of which they seem to be unaware, so that we do not 'bind their conscience.'

So learn what God has to say about dietary holiness and teach others the same.

Pride Pitfall

We are so eaten up with pride in this country that it is extremely hard for anyone to speak to anyone else about issues of sin in their lives. That is a formula for destruction, which is exactly what we are seeing in the Body of Christ... fatigue, sickness, obesity, etc.

"Pride goeth before destruction, and a haughty spirit before a fall." (Proverbs 16:18, KJV)

"... the most proud shall stumble and fall and no one will raise him up..." (Jeremiah 50:32, KJV)

"Ye stiffnecked and uncircumcised in heart and ears, ye do always resist the Holy Spirit..." (Acts 7:51, KJV)

In large part, we find ourselves 'stumbling' because of the pride in our heart. We are not open to correction, even from God, much less another Believer.

"... he that hardeneth his heart shall fall into mischief." (Proverbs 28:14, KJV)

'Mischief' is a good word to describe the dietary practices of God's people. Our pride keeps us in mischief, as it spiritually enables us to argue against any reason or truth presented to us, and to live in denial of any truth that would 'dare' require us to change our ways.

"For all that is in the world, the lust of the flesh, and the lust of the eyes, and the pride of life, is not of the Father, but is of the world." (I John 2:16, KJV)

Animal Anarchy – Acts 10:9-16

Of all the common misconceptions, I can most easily understand where the confusion may have come regarding God's commands concerning 'clean' and 'unclean' animals in Leviticus 11 and Deuteronomy 14 and what might appear to be the message in Acts 10:9-16. In summary, the Church has determined that Acts 10:9-16 proves that we can now eat unclean animal meats, thereby destroying the requirement for dietary holiness in our lives. I will explain why this is an incorrect interpretation.

God's message in Leviticus 11 and Deuteronomy 14 goes beyond clean and unclean animal meats. In these passages, God is demonstrating that what we eat matters to Him and that He does not want us to eat unhealthy things. So God's message here goes beyond unclean animal meats and applies to soda and donuts as well. Remember that soda and donuts did not exist at that time. There was nothing that Jesus could have done on the cross to change God's desire to bless us, and keep us from harm, through holy living, diet and health most certainly included.

Let's now carefully look at Acts 10:9-16.

"On the morrow, as they went on their journey, and drew nigh unto the city, Peter went up upon the housetop to pray about the sixth hour: And he became very hungry, and would have eaten: but while they made ready, he fell into a trance, And saw heaven opened, and a certain vessel descending unto him, as it had been a great sheet knit at the four corners, and let down to the earth: Wherein were all manner of fourfooted beasts of the earth, and wild beasts, and creeping things, and fowls of the air. And there came a voice to him, Rise, Peter; kill, and eat. But Peter said, Not so, Lord; for I have never eaten any thing that is common or unclean. And the voice spake unto him again the second time, What God hath cleansed, that call not thou common. This was done thrice: and the vessel was received up again into heaven." (Acts 10:9-16, KJV)

There are a number of points to make regarding this passage. One, this was a vision, not a literal event. Two, Peter never actually ate any of the unclean meats during the vision or after he woke up. And three, the purpose of this passage was to show Peter that under the New Covenant,

God saw Jews and Gentiles as one. It is also worth noting that there is no account in Scripture subsequent to this passage that shows God's people eating unclean animal meats.

The purpose of this passage was in no way for God to approve the consumption of unclean animal meats that would be harmful to our bodies. And as we saw before, the application of unclean animal meats in Leviticus 11 and Deuteronomy 14 extends to all substances that are unhealthy for us, soda and donuts, for example.

But why would God have used such a confusing example to teach us that the Gentiles and Jews were now one? Let's consider another example that is equally confusing. God had once told Abraham to sacrifice his son, Isaac. Now, this is just as confusing. How could God ask Abraham to kill an innocent person? How could God possibly okay murder?

I cannot understand why it is okay for God to direct someone to seemingly 'sin' in an effort for Him to test their faith or teach them something, nevertheless, that is exactly what God has done in these two examples. But in both of these examples we must recognize that God never actually allowed the sinful consumption of those unclean animals or the sinful murder of an innocent person. Regardless of either Peter's or Abraham's response, Peter would have never been allowed to physically eat of the unclean animals and Abraham would have never been allowed to murder Isaac.

If someone wants to argue that Peter's vision was God's way of telling us that unclean meats (unhealthy eating) are now okay to eat, then they will also have to argue that the story of Abraham and Isaac is God's way of telling us that murder is okay.

I try to stay away from 'man's wisdom' as much as possible, as it usually harms more than helps. But I do believe that any 'good science' works to only prove out what the Bible has said all along. This is a very good application for some good science.

If you took the animals listed in Leviticus 11 and Deuteronomy 14, and sorted them on a 'toxicity scale,' which is exactly what scientists have done, you would see that deer, chicken, beef, tuna and bass are at the bottom of the toxicity scale (good for you). You will also see that pork, catfish, crab, and shrimp are at the very top of the toxicity scale (bad for you). Obviously, nothing that Jesus did on the cross affected the chemical makeup of clean and unclean animal meats, and their positive or negative effects on our bodies.

Unique Undoing

What I have termed Unique Undoing is one of those extremely effective methods by which Satan can keep us from focusing on and applying God's dietary truths to our lives. It is commonly stated that 'we are all different' whenever a discussion about diet comes up. In so doing, any wisdom of God on the matter just seems to be dismissed because 'what is right for you may not be right for me.'

Although God has certainly made each of us 'unique,' His principles for living are anything but unique to the individual. God's principles are the same yesterday, today, and tomorrow, and they apply to all of us equally. Junk non-foods like refined sugars damage all our bodies. Fruits and vegetables are nutritious and healing for all our bodies.

So often, when someone is talking about a medical condition they are struggling with, they will say that they are 'on a special diet.' There is only One diet, and that is God's diet. The only Biblically supported 'special diet' is a fast. Fasting is an essential component for growth and healing in spirit, soul, and body. Fasting is beyond the scope of this book; however, I will point you to Isaiah 58:6-12 to learn more about the benefits of fasting.

Another problem with these 'special diets' is that they are short-term. A proper and righteous diet (God's diet) is not a temporary fix, but a way of life that leads to abundance in physical health. There are no 'quick fixes' in God's economy. God will not be mocked. Our sins will find us out.

"… be sure that your sin will find you out." (Numbers 32:23, KJV)

"Be not deceived; God is not mocked; for whatsoever a man soweth, that shall he also reap." (Galatians 6:7, KJV)

I will say that in the case of certain degenerative conditions, some foods, even God's foods, have a reaction that is very unpleasant. I know of one individual whose colon would flare up in intense pain and discomfort for several weeks every six months or so. If he were to eat a salad during those inflamed periods, especially one with carrots in it, he would suffer quite severely.

So what did he eat to avoid the discomfort of such roughage? He avoided salads for sure, but he was also sure to continue eating junk non-foods that didn't 'seem' to irritate his inflamed condition. These included soda, white breads, and pastries, the very substances that were the cause of his problem to begin with. If healthy foods irritated his colon during this time, the best solution for him would have been to fast.

"For as the heavens are higher than the earth, so are my ways higher than your ways, and my thoughts than your thoughts." (Isaiah 55:9, KJV)

Although salads might have been inappropriate for the few weeks his condition was inflamed, he did not eat them the six months or so he had off between episodes either. I tried to tell him that if he would eat more vegetables and fruits during the off periods, he might find that the occurrence of his episodes would disappear completely.

Did he listen to the wisdom of God that I tried to impart to him? Did he give up his gallon of soda a day (not an exaggeration – he drank soda like water) or his white, bleached bread? Did he give up his Debbie Cakes? Did he eat vegetables and fruits when his condition was not inflamed? No he didn't. About a year after my last conversation with him in this regard he had several feet of his colon removed, a victim of dietary deception.

"A prudent man foreseeth the evil, and hideth himself, but the simple pass on and are punished." (Proverbs 22:3, KJV)

This fellow reminds me of another encounter I had with such dietary deception. Years ago, a co-worker of mine was mentioning that her husband was having some health problems. Among other things, I asked her if he ate vegetables, salads, and the like. She indicated that he was a 'meat and potatoes' man. He would say that 'salads are for rabbits.' Well, he was suffering with colon cancer. I have not heard of too many wild rabbits coming down with colon cancer.

"...I am the Lord thy God, which teacheth thee to profit, which leadeth thee by the way that thou shouldest go. O that thou hadst hearkened to my commandments!..." (Isaiah 48:17-18, KJV)

Fallen Fiasco

Yes, we do live in a fallen world. But even within our fallen world, God has given us His instruction book, the Bible, and His guide, the Holy Spirit, to ensure our spiritual, emotional, and physical welfare. Be that as it may, many will use the excuse that because we live in a fallen world we have no choice but to give in to the perverted non-foods produced.

Many would argue that we should give in to and endure whatever evils happen to come via the world's system, because after all, we are 'victims of a fallen world.' We've already talked about lifespan. But it is worth mentioning here as well. Even in this fallen world, God has still provided the instructions to enable an obedient people to live 120 years (Genesis 6:3). And we have already shown that the lifespan we are seeing today, 70 to 80 years, is that of a sinful people (Psalm 90:7-12). This reality has nothing to do with the 'fallen world.' This reality has to do with disobedience. We are not 'victims' in this regard.

If you choose soda over water, you are not a victim of a fallen world. You have chosen to partake in the sins of a fallen world. If you choose pastries over fruit, you are not a victim of a fallen world. You have chosen to partake in the sins of a fallen world. If you choose refined sugar over honey, you are not a victim of a fallen world. You have chosen to partake in the sins of a fallen world. If you feed your children candy instead of fruit, you are not a victim of a fallen world. You have chosen to partake in the sins of a fallen world. When you choose to bake a bunch of cookies for someone who is having a hard time instead of giving them a hug or words of comfort from the Scriptures, you are not a victim of a fallen world. You have chosen to partake in the sins of a fallen world.

I think you get the picture.

Latter License – I Timothy 4:1-5

"Now the Spirit speaketh expressly, that in the latter times some shall depart from the faith, giving heed to seducing spirits, and doctrines of devils: Speaking lies in hypocrisy; having their conscience seared with a hot iron; Forbidding to marry, and commanding to abstain from meats, which God hath created to be received with thanksgiving of them which believe and know the truth. For every creature of God is good, and nothing to be refused, if it be received with thanksgiving: For it is sanctified by the word of God and prayer." (I Timothy 4:1-5, KJV)

I can see how someone could read this passage and try to use it to dismiss this entire book. It might seem to communicate that to command that God's people abstain from unclean meats is an evil of the latter days. But that is not what this passage is saying here.

For starters, this verse is referencing the directives that will come from those who have departed from the faith and have given heed to seducing spirits and doctrines of devils. I hope I don't have to tell you that this doesn't describe me.

Second, this 'abstain from meats' text is in tandem with 'forbidding to marry.' I am certainly not suggesting that people should no longer marry, in this book and any other book I might write. So this passage is applicable to a much broader context of spiritual deception and satanic doctrine.

Third, the 'meats' it's talking about are not unclean meats, but rather clean meats, the meats that 'God hath created to be received.' God never created the unclean meats to be received as food. The 'meats' spoken of here are clean meats, which relative to consumption, is 'every creature of God.' Unclean meats are not 'creatures of God' for consumption.

And fourth, any clean meats that might have been formally sacrificed to idols, or been part of any spiritually deprived ceremony, are sanctified (set apart and still valuable for nourishment) as God's Word tells us in I Corinthians 10. There is no 'voodoo hex' that man can put on God's foods that will alter the ability of that food to nourish our bodies. Satan doesn't have the power to do that.

Reckless Romans – Romans 6:13-15

Without a doubt, the book of Romans, as a whole, is the most misinterpreted book in the Bible, most especially as it applies to the subject of this book. We have already looked at a couple of passages in Romans that have been misinterpreted to support dietary deception. Let's take a look at yet another, Romans 6:13-15.

"Neither yield ye your members as instruments of unrighteousness unto sin: but yield yourselves unto God, as those that are alive from the dead, and your members as instruments of righteousness unto God. For sin shall not have dominion over you: for ye are not under the law, but under grace. What then? shall we sin, because we are not under the law, but under grace? God forbid." (Romans 6:13-15, KJV)

The generally accepted take-away from this passage is that we are no longer responsible to answer to any Old Testament law, Leviticus 11 concerning clean and unclean animal meats, for example. Nothing could be further from the truth. Let's break down this passage verse by verse to reveal its true meaning.

Verse 13) Neither yield ye your members as instruments of unrighteousness unto sin: but yield yourselves unto God, as those that are alive from the dead, and your members as instruments of righteousness unto God.
This passage begins with an encouragement to Believers to live our lives righteously.

Verse 14) For sin shall not have dominion over you: for ye are not under the law, but under grace.
We are then told that sin should not have dominion over us (i.e. we should live righteously). We should be able to live righteously, not because our salvation is by the law (under the law), but because our salvation is now by grace (under grace). Note the difference between righteous, or holy, living noted in Verse 13 compared with the topic of salvation by grace in Verse 14.

Verse 15) What then? shall we sin, because we are not under the law, but under grace? God forbid.
Although our salvation is by grace, and grace alone (we are not saved by the law / under the law), yet our obedience to the law is still an issue of obedience verses sin, an issue of righteous living.

This passage defines or addresses legalism. Legalism would argue that we could be saved by the law through righteous living (under the law). This is not the case as it points out. We can only be saved by grace (under grace), and not by works or by the law. But at the same time, although we are under grace in terms of salvation, God still has a standard for holy living upon our lives as defined by the law, the deviation from which is sin.

I am not saying that the ceremonial and sacrificial components of the Old Testament apply to us today. The purpose of the ceremonial and sacrificial components was to point towards the coming Messiah and to provide us with access to God. Jesus' coming completed, brought to fruition, the purpose of those practices. Jesus was the ultimate and final sacrifice. We are certainly not 'under the law' in the sense that we are required to perform animal sacrifices for our sins, nor do we have to go through the high priest to access God.

But for the physical laws concerning diet and cleanliness, for example, there should be no doubt that these would apply to us as equally today as they did 4,000 years ago. The evil fruit of our turning away from those laws substantially supports that. There is nothing Jesus could have done on the cross, or would have wanted to accomplish on the cross, that would have freed us to live life in an unrighteousness and destructive manner (dietary deception). A lack of dietary holiness will not make us a light on a hill, will not put us above all the nations, and will not make us a witness of God's wisdom and power to the rest of the world.

Right Romans – Romans 3:31

Many passages in Romans tend to be quite confusing and open to misinterpretation, as you have already seen. But Romans 3:31 succinctly clarifies the matter of whether or not God's dietary directives still apply to us today. I will quote Romans 3:31 from both the King James Version and The Message to offer the greatest level of clarity possible in this case.

"Do we then make void the law through faith? God forbid: yea, we establish the law." (Romans 3:31, KJV)

"But by shifting our focus from what we do to what God does, don't we cancel out all our careful keeping of the rules and ways God commanded? Not at all.

What happens, in fact, is that by putting that entire way of life in its proper place, we confirm it." (Romans 3:31, MSG, BibleGateway.com)

No further comment necessary.

Concession Confusion – Acts 15

In Acts 15 we have some text that offers some room for confusion. Most have concluded that Acts 15 tells us that we can eat anything we want, with the exception of a few basic rules. But between digging deeper into what is being communicated in Acts 15, and keeping in mind all of the truths of Scripture we have covered up until now, I think you should be able to see that Acts 15 does not overturn God's standard for holiness in the area of diet. You will see that what is being addressed in Acts 15 includes legalism, salvation by grace alone, and concessions between the Jews and Gentiles regarding certain 'offend thy brother' types of practices similar to what we discussed earlier in I Corinthians 10.

I won't list the entire chapter, but only those verses most applicable to our discussion.

"1)   And certain men which came down from Judea taught the brethren, and said, Except ye be circumcised after the manner of Moses, ye cannot be saved.

2)   When therefore Paul and Barnabas had no small dissension and disputation with them, they determined that Paul and Barnabas, and certain other of them, should go up to Jerusalem unto the apostles and elders about this question.

5)   But there rose up certain of the sect of the Pharisees which believed saying, That it was needful to circumcise them, and to command them to keep the law of Moses.

6)   And the apostles and elders came together for to consider of this matter.

7)   And when there had been much disputing, Peter rose up, and said unto them, Men and brethren, ye know how that a good while ago God made choice among us, that the Gentiles by my mouth should hear the word of the gospel, and believe.

8) *And God, which knoweth the hearts, bare them witness, giving them the Holy Ghost, even as he did unto us;*

9) *And put no difference between us and them, purifying their hearts by faith.*

10) *Now therefore why tempt ye God, to put a yoke upon the neck of the disciples, which neither our fathers nor we were able to bear?*

11) *But we believe that through the grace of the Lord Jesus Christ we shall be saved, even as they.*

23) *And they wrote letters by them after this manner; The apostles and elders and brethren send greeting unto the brethren which are of the Gentiles in Antioch and Syria and Cilicia.*

24) *Forasmuch as we have heard that certain which went out from us have troubled you with words, subverting your souls, saying, Ye must be circumcised, and keep the law: to whom we gave no such commandment:*

28) *For it seemed good to the Holy Ghost, and to us, to lay upon you no greater burden than these necessary things;*

29) *That ye abstain from meats offered to idols, and from blood, and from things strangled, and from fornication: from which if ye keep yourselves, ye shall do well, Fare ye well.*

31) *Which when they had read, they rejoiced for the consolation." (Portions of Acts 15:1-31, KJV)*

Okay, you know the drill. Let's carefully unpack these verses to get a clear understanding of what is being said here.

Verse 1) And certain men which came down from Judea taught the brethren, and said, Except ye be circumcised after the manner of Moses, ye cannot be saved.

Right off the bat, we see that the issue of legalism is at hand. These 'certain men' tried to tell God's people that you cannot be saved unless you are circumcised. This is a classic example of legalism, attaching any requirement to salvation by grace and grace alone.

Verse 2) When therefore Paul and Barnabas had no small dissension and disputation with them, they determined that Paul and Barnabas, and certain other of them, should go up to Jerusalem unto the apostles and elders about this question.

Paul obviously had a major issue with this legalistic view.

Verse 5) But there rose up certain of the sect of the Pharisees which believed saying, That it was needful to circumcise them, and to command them to keep the law of Moses.

It looks like we have another group that wants God's people to believe that circumcision and adherence to the law of Moses is required for salvation. Of course, these are not. To contend in this way is legalism. That being said, this does not mean that the law of Moses regarding diet and health is no longer a component of holy living. But holy living is not what is being addressed here. Salvation, or requirements for salvation (legalism), is the focus.

Verse 6) And the apostles and elders came together for to consider of this matter.

Verse 7) And when there had been much disputing, Peter rose up, and said unto them, Men and brethren, ye know how that a good while ago God made choice among us, that the Gentiles by my mouth should hear the word of the gospel, and believe.

Verse 8) And God, which knoweth the hearts, bare them witness, giving them the Holy Ghost, even as he did unto us;

Verse 9) And put no difference between us and them, purifying their hearts by faith.

The point is made that salvation is by faith, not works and holy living.

Verse 10) Now therefore why tempt ye God, to put a yoke upon the neck of the disciples, which neither our fathers nor we were able to bear?
With the exception of Jesus Christ, Who walked in perfect dietary holiness, no other person has been able to perfectly live out the holy standards of the law. Consequently, no person could ever earn salvation through perfect obedience to the law. It is only by grace that any of us could be saved.

Verse 11) But we believe that through the grace of the Lord Jesus Christ we shall be saved, even as they.
The emphasis here is that both the Jews and the Gentiles can be saved by faith through grace, not by any works or requirements one group lays upon the other. This settles the whole legalism argument once and for all, as well as nullifies the distinction between Jew and Gentile.

Verse 23) And they wrote letters by them after this manner; The apostles and elders and brethren send greeting unto the brethren which are of the Gentiles in Antioch and Syria and Cilicia.

Verse 24) Forasmuch as we have heard that certain which went out from us have troubled you with words, subverting your souls, saying, Ye must be circumcised, and keep the law: to whom we gave no such commandment:
Again, salvation is not determined by circumcision or keeping the law. Holy living is not what is being addressed here.

Verse 28) For it seemed good to the Holy Ghost, and to us, to lay upon you no greater burden than these necessary things;

Verse 29) That ye abstain from meats offered to idols, and from blood, and from things strangled, and from fornication: from which if ye keep yourselves, ye shall do well, Fare ye well.

'abstain from meats offered to idols' – As we discussed in I Corinthians 10, those 'weak in faith' took issue with the consumption of foods formally sacrificed to idols, while those 'strong in faith' did not. But in an effort to ease the tensions, the request was made that everyone abstain from any foods formally sacrificed to idols in order to ensure no one was offended either way.

'abstain from blood' – Leviticus 7:26 tells us that we should not eat the blood of an animal. Modern science shows why this is a good practice. Although nutrients are transported throughout the body by way of the blood, toxins are also dumped from the body into the bloodstream for eventual elimination. Therefore, for example, although the meat of a cow is clean from a toxicity standpoint, its blood is unclean/toxic. I really don't know why this stipulation needed to be added amongst the 'concessions,' being an understood component of holy living.

'abstain from things strangled' – Again, modern science has been able to offer some insight into why this is a good practice. When an animal is given time to struggle and suffer during the death process, such as what is possible through strangulation, hormones and toxins are distributed into the animal's musculature as part of the emergency response process. This event, from a health standpoint, increases the toxicity levels of the meat we might consume.

'abstain from fornication' – In Romans 6 we saw that salvation by grace does not give us license to sin. Although avoidance of sexual sin should have been an understood requirement for holy living by all, I can only assume that some decided to inappropriately use grace to justify or enable their fleshly desires in this way.

This verse and passage in no way indicates that unclean meats (and unhealthy junk non-foods by principle) are now okay for consumption.

It was understood by all, Jew and Gentile alike, that the consumption of unclean meats constituted sin, although not a requirement for salvation. That is why this issue is not part of the compromise to ease the tensions in the congregation.

Verse 31) Which when they had read, they rejoiced for the consolation.
These restrictions were highlighted in an effort to ease the tensions in the congregation, to console those of differing views on what was and was not okay to do. In no way was this small list of restrictions meant to constitute all that was required of God's people to live holy before God. This is obvious because nothing is mentioned regarding murder, theft, unclean animal meats, or any other area of holy living that God is concerned about.

Love Lunacy

The biggest promoters of the deviation from dietary holiness in the Church are often the most well-meaning. In adult Sunday-school classes a member that desires to serve others might bring donuts to class. Those that are sick or hurting in some way are brought pastries and desserts by well-meaning members of the congregation. Children are rewarded with candy for learning Bible verses. Both the giver and the receiver take this as an expression of 'love,' misguided as it may be.

Although their heart's intent is good, their actions constitute an evil exercised against the very ones they are trying to love. The way in which these well-meaning people are trying to serve others is no different than someone bringing beer and cigarettes to church in an effort to provide everyone with a more festive worship experience. The intent may be good, but the path is bad, even sinful. There are better ways to love others than by working to destroy their health, creating addictive and unhealthy eating patterns in their lives, and keeping them from their ideal body weight.

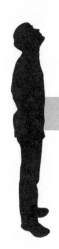
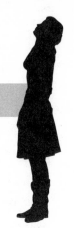

Chapter 23

The Sin Proof – A Study of Refined Sugars

Until we can determine that a particular activity is addressed in the Bible as a matter of holy living we cannot say that it represents an issue of obedience verses sin. If the Bible does point to an activity as a matter of holy living (do not lie, for example) then we can claim that it represents an issue of obedience verses sin. Otherwise, the activity does not represent an issue of obedience verses sin and is only a matter of preference.

In this chapter we will determine whether the consumption of, or abstinence from, refined sugars is a matter of preference or if it is a matter of holy living, representing an issue of obedience verses sin. If I am unable to determine that the abstinence from refined sugars is a Biblically supported standard for holy living on our lives, representing an issue of obedience verses sin, then this book should be tossed into the trash can.

This study could have just as easily been based on refined flours, hydrogenated oils, or any other man-made product that we might consume that is unhealthy for our bodies. But I thought refined sugars would be a category most familiar to everyone. The types of substances that contain significant amounts of refined sugars include packets/bags of refined sugar of course, soda, pastries, cookies, syrups and jellies, and candy, for example.

We saw in our study of Leviticus 11 and Deuteronomy 14, where

God distinguished between clean and unclean animal meats, that His standard for holy living included a concern about what we ate and our health. We observed that God demonstrated that He did not want us to put anything in our bodies that is harmful.

Through modern science, it has been made vividly clear that the clean animals have low toxicity levels and the unclean animals have high toxicity levels. So we know that God's differentiation between clean and unclean was based on His concern for our physical well-being. And similarly, we also know that refined sugars are harmful to our bodies.

We also determined that the point of these passages was not limited to animal meats alone, but to anything we might eat, keeping in mind that if refined sugars, for example, had existed at that time, the Bible would have directly addressed them as well.

By the way, for those who would argue that this dietary requirement was only applicable to those people at that time, they need only go to Genesis 7 to see this belief dismissed. It is in Genesis 7 that God directs Noah to gather a certain number of clean and unclean animals. Long before the time of Leviticus 11 and Deuteronomy 14, from the beginning, there was an understanding that there were clean and unclean animals. As we saw earlier, this did not impact our diets until after the world flood when God directed man to begin eating animals.

The American Heritage Dictionary defines evil as follows: 'Evil – … Causing ruin, injury, or pain; harmful. Characterized by or indicating future misfortune… something that causes harm, misfortune, or destruction… something that is the cause or source of suffering, injury, or destruction.' I am not trying to base this proof on what the American Heritage Dictionary has to say about the matter, but I think we can all agree that this would be a Biblically supported list of the characteristics of sin / evil.

Do refined sugars cause ruin in our health and to our emotions through the spirit-emotion-body connection? Yes.

229

Do refined sugars cause injury and pain to our bodies (consider diabetes and weight gain, for example)? Yes.

Do refined sugars harm our bodies? Yes.

Does the consumption of refined sugars lead to future misfortune (diabetes and weight gain, for example)? Yes.

Does all of Scripture tell us that God wants to direct our lives in ways (holy living) that keep us from harm? Yes.

Does the manufacture of refined sugars constitute a chemical perversion of God's designed foods? Yes

Does the poor health created by refined sugars hinder our ability to better serve God and others? Yes

Does the consumption of refined sugars support the objectives of Satan in our lives, while thwarting the desires of God for our lives? Yes

Does the consumption of refined sugars represent a conformation to the ways of this world, as opposed to the ways of God? Yes

Does the effect of refined sugars on our spirits, souls, and bodies violate the very character, nature, and desires of a loving God? Yes

Does the consumption of refined sugars constitute a 'sowing to the flesh', which is destructive, as opposed to a 'sowing to the Spirit', which produces life? Yes

We also saw earlier that to argue that God cared about our physical health and required a holy standard for our dietary practices before Jesus came, but then 'freed us' to harm ourselves through unhealthy dietary practices and enslave us to substances like refined sugar after Jesus came, is preposterous.

"Let your light so shine before men, that they may see your good works, and glorify your Father which is in Heaven. Think not that I am come to destroy the law, or the prophets: I am not come to destroy, but to fulfill." (Matthew 5:16-18, KJV)

Does a people struggling with fatigue, sickness, and obesity 'shine a light before all men of their good works?' No. Is this glorifying to God? No.

There are few evils visited upon mankind as destructive to spirit, soul, and body as refined sugars. Refined sugars contribute to an addictive nature that is destructive spiritually and emotionally, as well as physically. It is a known scientific fact that refined sugars are the primary culprit in the development of the degenerative conditions of obesity, diabetes, cancer, cardiovascular disease, osteoporosis, etc.

Refined sugars create violent blood sugar changes that work to destroy the pancreas, adrenals, and thyroid over time. Refined sugars disrupt the body's alkaline and mineral balances within the blood. Refined sugars steal nutrients from the body, rather than provide nutrients. Refined sugars are acidic to the body, while the body functions best in an alkaline state. And refined sugars are quickly converted into excess fat.

Who is it that desires to harm us in this way? Who is the Angel of Light seeking to deceive both the world and the Believer? Who could possibly be the author of something as destructive as refined sugars? Who is that thief? Is it not Satan?

"The thief cometh not, but for to steal, and to kill, and to destroy..." (John 10:10, KJV)

Could refined sugars be God's will for our lives, with all the sorrow that it has brought upon mankind, upon you? No.

"The blessing of the Lord maketh rich, and he addeth no sorrow with it." (Proverbs 10:22, KJV)

"For I know the thoughts that I think toward you, saith the Lord, thoughts of peace, and not of evil…" (Jeremiah 29:11, KJV)

Did Jesus come to give us an abundant life? Yes. Is the degenerative health and excess weight caused by refined sugars part of an abundant life? No.

"…I am come that they might have life, and that they might have it more abundantly." (John 10:10, KJV)

Have refined sugars brought forth good fruit in your life? No.

"For a good tree bringeth not forth corrupt fruit, neither doth a corrupt tree bring forth good fruit, for every tree is known by his own fruit…" (Luke 6:43-44, KJV)

Folks, if it looks like a duck, walks like a duck, and sounds like a duck, it just might be a duck. If this book and this chapter aren't enough to convince you that refined sugars are an evil perversion of what God would have to be food for us, and that to believe otherwise doesn't constitute dietary deception, I would conclude that you do not have 'ears to hear.'

"… he that hath ears to hear, let him hear." (Luke 8:8, KJV)

"For every one that doeth evil hateth the light, neither cometh to the light, lest his deeds should be reproved." (John 3:20, KJV)

I want to encourage you to read *Sugar Blues* by William Dufty. In his book Dufty does a fantastic job of demonstrating the evils of refined sugars, its history being truly remarkable. Refined sugar was the cause of wars, slavery, the fall of entire countries, degenerative diseases, food refinement advances, and it even changed the Church.

I love this excerpt from an article by Leonard Haimes, M.D; entitled *Refined Sugar – Gradual Suicide*. He could not be any more accurate.

'It's as if the devil sat down and listed all the criteria of a substance that man could use to destroy himself. It would have to be pleasing to the eye and taste, be pure white and easily available, and appeal to all the people of this world. The destroying effect would have to be subtle and take such a long time that very few would realize what was happening until it was too late. The cruelest criteria of all is it would have to be supported and distributed by the kindest, well-meaning people to the most innocent people.'

We must be willing to 'declare our iniquity' as David exclaimed in Psalms 38:18. We must 'not cover our sins' as Solomon stated in Proverbs 28:13. We can no longer 'pervert our way and forget the Lord our God' as Jeremiah protested in Jeremiah 3:21-22. We must 'confess our sinfulness' before we can experience deliverance as John urges in I John 1:9. In the context of diet and health, confess means that you 'agree with God' and 'admit to God' that your ways are wrong, sinful, and destructive, and that God's Weigh is right, holy, and beneficial.

"For I will declare mine iniquity; I will be sorry for my sin." (Psalm 38:18, KJV)

"He that covereth his sins shall not prosper: but whoso confesseth and forsaketh them shall have mercy." (Proverbs 28:13)

"... *they have perverted their way, and they have forgotten the Lord their God. Return, ye backsliding children, and I will heal your backslidings...*" (*Jeremiah 3:21-22, KJV*)

"*If we confess our sins, he is faithful and just to forgive us our sins, and to cleanse us from all unrighteousness.*" (*I John 1:9, KJV*)

Without the recognition of sin, there can be no acknowledgement of sin. Without the acknowledgment of sin, there can be no confession of sin. Without the confession of sin, there can be no deliverance from sin. Without deliverance from sin, there can be no deliverance from the consequences of sin. This is how dietary deception has kept you from your ideal body weight.

Does the consumption of refined sugars constitute sin? I think this chapter should have successfully demonstrated the evil that refined sugars truly are.

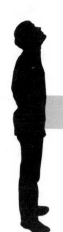
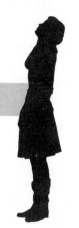

Chapter 24

Dietary Deception & Dietary Holiness Fully Defined

Throughout this book I have referred to the terms dietary deception and dietary holiness. Although the meaning of these two terms was implied and applied in the text along the way, I want to define them very clearly and extensively for you here.

I had initially planned to include this chapter early on in the book, right after the Introduction. But after further consideration I determined that you might not be ready to receive these Biblical insights until after you had read the rest of the book. For most, I think that to go from thinking like the rest of the Church regarding diet and health to seeing dietary deception and dietary holiness unveiled in such a direct, hard-hitting way would have been too big a jump to make.

Hang on tight. This is some very heavy stuff. Your flesh will not like it. Your carnal nature will fight tooth and nail against it. And unfortunately, the Church has worked against it. But the Holy Spirit working within you will resonate with it. And by now you are ready for it. So here we go...

Dietary deception is made up of a number of beliefs and characteristics. These include...

1) Satan's deception of God's people into supporting the view that the perversion of God's created foods, and the deviation from His

explicit commands for our dietary practices as outlined in the Bible, in quality and quantity, do not constitute sin, despite the damage well known to be exacted upon our bodies, the very bodies that are no longer our own, having been purchased by God through Jesus Christ.

2) Rather, as motivated by their fallen, fleshly nature, God's people preferring to argue that these behaviors are part of the Believer's 'freedoms in Christ' or to label such a standard for righteousness upon their lives as 'legalistic,' regardless of the evil fruit produced by these evil works.

3) All the while, God's people refusing to ever search the Scriptures and seek God on the matter for themselves, failing to learn that what we eat does matter to God, thereby enabling them to maintain their desired position in darkness, far away from any light of God that might be shown upon their sinful hearts, which would surely lead to a call for death to self and a departure from the dietary patterns of this world.

4) These being spiritual requirements God's people already know they are unwilling to address. Rather, God's people choosing to follow the world in search for some magic pill or magic formula for health that would overcome the consequences of their sinful ways, the Church, in effect, determining that their diets are 'off-limits' to God.

5) The leadership of the Church refusing to offend anyone with the harder truths of God's Word, excusing their behavior as being 'loving,' while in reality, functioning as an essential accomplice to the works of Satan within the Body of Christ in this regard. The leadership of the Church knowing it is not prepared spiritually and in wisdom to

either communicate the Word of God concerning diet and health, nor prepared spiritually to walk in obedience themselves.

6) God's people not recognizing that successful living is the greatest evangelical tool available to us through the wisdom and power of God's Word, the achievement of health and our ideal body weight constituting the perfect venue whereby we can glorify God, attracting the world to Him.

7) Dietary deception represents Biblical heresy relative to the truths and commands of God's Word concerning diet and health, along with the violation of a variety of other spiritual principles along the way.

By contrast, dietary holiness is the polar opposite of dietary deception in each belief and characteristic...

1) God's people supporting the view that the perversion of God's created foods, and the deviation from His explicit commands for our dietary practices as outlined in the Bible, in quality and quantity, constitutes sin, recognizing that our bodies are no longer our own, not to be treated in any manner we see fit, having been purchased by God through Jesus Christ.

2) God's people arguing that their freedoms in Christ in no way give license to the free destruction of their bodies, understanding that although this is not a requirement for salvation, which would make it legalism, but that it is rather a component of righteous living, one that will provide good fruit in their lives.

3) God's people searching the Scriptures and seeking God on the matter for themselves, learning that what we eat does matter to

God, thereby enabling them to depart from the dietary patterns of the world and to walk in righteousness, freedom, and victory.

4) These being spiritual requirements God's people are willing to address. God's people choosing not to follow the world in search for some magic pill or magic formula for health that would overcome the consequences of their sinful ways, the Church determining that their diets are God's to direct and control.

5) The leadership of the Church willingly teaching these harder truths of God's Word, in 'tough love,' functioning as an essential tool to edify the Body of Christ in this regard. The leadership of the Church knowing it must be prepared spiritually and in wisdom to communicate the Word of God concerning diet and health, and must be prepared to walk in obedience themselves.

6) God's people recognizing that successful living is the greatest evangelical tool available to us through the wisdom and power of God's Word, the achievement of health and our ideal body weight constituting the perfect venue whereby we can glorify God, attracting the world to Him.

7) Dietary holiness represents an understanding of the Biblical truths and commands of God's Word concerning diet and health, along with their impact on all areas of the Christian walk.

If the rest of the book hasn't already convinced you of the Biblical realities of dietary deception and dietary holiness then I don't know what else to say.

In many ways, I wish all this wasn't true. I had rather be able to live my life any way that I wanted to, enjoy good fruit from all my actions, and it all be found pleasing to God. But that just isn't reality. The reality is that if you and I live our lives any way we want we will incur bad fruit from our actions, and God will not be pleased.

Look at where you are right now. Does your current reality, the fruit of controlling your own actions in the area of diet and health, not support this? You know it does. That gnawing in your gut is the Holy Spirit working to reveal this to you.

Throughout this book I trust that the Biblical realities of dietary deception and dietary holiness have already become clear to you. I hope this chapter has only worked to help wrap these terms and their application into a tight package and summary for you.

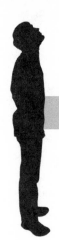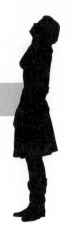

Chapter 25

How Does All This Play Out in the Real World?

Here you are. You have been tucked away in a quiet, cozy, protected room reading this book. You are fully sold on the Biblical principles concerning diet and health outlined herein. Now what?

I realize that you won't take more than a few steps out of that room before you begin to wonder how you are supposed to pull this off in the real world. After all, concerning diet and health, sin is everywhere; in your home, in your community, and even in your church.

The very first people you walk by, your spouse and your children, may not be happy and supportive of your new-found Biblical enlightenment. They will continue to demand the same junk non-foods to which they have always been accustomed. And even if you refuse to partake yourself they may choose to continue with their sinful eating practices right in front of you. If both you and your spouse have struggled in this area, your spouse may even resent you for 'leaving them behind.' They may never verbalize it in those words, but that may be how they are made to feel.

How do you handle this situation? I hope that after reading this book you have learned that God's Word has the answers to all of our tough life questions. Case in point...

"If any man come to me, and hate not his father, and mother, and wife, and

children, and brethren, and sisters, yea, and his own life also, he cannot be my disciple." (Luke 14:26, KJV)

I haven't heard anyone interpret this verse correctly yet. The best anyone has offered in the way of interpretation is that compared to how much we love God how much we love our family would look like hate. That is incorrect.

For starters, we know that God is not calling us to hate anyone in the way we tend to think of hate. We all know that God calls us to love one another. So why the confusing contradiction?

What this verse is talking about is 'prioritization.' This verse calls God's people to prioritize His commandments and desires over the desires of our families. 'Hating' our family, in this context, means that if your family wants you to sell illegal drugs, for example, you will refuse, thereby prioritizing the desires of God for your life (loving God) over the desires of others for your life (hating your family).

So let's apply this verse to your situation. You have a spouse and children, or friends and colleagues, who demand that you partake in their sinful dietary practices. You know that avoiding that chocolate cake and soda is God's will for your life. What do you do? You say 'no.' And by saying 'no' you have loved God and hated your spouse, children, friends, and colleagues. That is not an easy thing to do, but that is exactly what God has called you to do. You will have to refuse to purchase, cook, and provide the junk non-foods they may demand, and you must certainly refuse to partake with them.

Your friends, co-workers, and fellow Believers at church may be equally upset and non-supportive. Not only will these people be upset with you, but they may even think you have joined some kind of cult. Just tell them, 'I now realize that my body is God's. I have no right to destroy it with harmful substances.' And then live out your life in front of them in obedience to Luke 14:26.

But don't see this as a problem, but rather an opportunity. This is a great opportunity for you to set an example for those who would discourage you or not agree with you. Let them see you drop 25, 50, 75, 100+ pounds, more energetic with each passing day, and then dare to challenge the truths of Scripture concerning diet and health, and the wisdom and power of God available to His people.

You show them. They then will get on board and show the rest of the church. And your church then will get on board and show the Body of Christ in your community. And the Body of Christ in your community then will get on board, etc. In that process there will be a growing swell of publicity within the world that something incredible is happening in the Church. And the world will want to know what we are doing differently, why we are doing it differently, and who told us to do it differently. We can then share with them the wisdom and power of God that can save their temporal bodies, and more importantly, share with them the wisdom and power of God that can save their eternal souls. You need to catch that vision for the Church and the world.

I would love to tell you that I have it all 100% worked out in my own home. But things still slip through. The kids get candy at church, one of the biggest pushers of sinful junk non-foods around. There are birthday parties and celebrations that make keeping everyone in line extremely difficult. But just like you can't keep your children from hearing things you don't want them to hear, you won't be able to always keep your children from eating things they shouldn't eat. It is simply another component of the growth process for them and the parenting process for you.

When someone asks me if my child can have a donut or some candy, I will often respond 'No thank you. I don't want my child to develop diabetes.' I think we should take every opportunity to direct others' attention to the consequences ahead of sin in the area of diet and health, especially when such drugs are pushed at our children.

But it isn't all bad and perpetually uphill. You will be surprised how quickly young children catch on to eating healthy. My seven year-old son recently walked up to a basket full of candy at the grocery store and said

'Yuk. Look Dad at all that sugary candy.' I have had child-care workers show their amazement when they see my kids eating salad, nuts/seeds, and fruit for snacks and meals instead of Goldfish, Cheerios, mac-n-cheese, chicken nuggets, and pastries.

As with any area of parenting, raising your children to live holy lives will occur by example, by direction, and by boundaries. I don't want my children to eat a donut any more than I want them to say curse words, be rude to someone, or fail to do their share of the work. It is all the same. I would contend that 'dietary parenting' is one of the most important areas of instruction when it comes to holy living.

Another difficulty you will face in the 'real world' is completely avoiding refined sugars, refined flours, and hydrogenated oils, for example, despite your greatest efforts. You will not be able to do so completely. You have to do the best you can. Unfortunately, there will be traces of these substances in a great number of 'relatively healthy' things you might have available to you to eat.

If you are unable to eat a salad because you only have ranch dressing available to you, I would encourage you to eat the salad with the ranch dressing. That is the best you can do in that situation. We live in a real world full of sin and man's ways. We can't change that in the short-term, but as a Church we should begin demanding 100% holy foods from manufacturers. They will answer to us once they see how much of their income comes from the Christian community.

I don't believe God expects us to turn dietary holiness into a full-time job, which is exactly what it would be if we demanded absolute perfection from ourselves. I think there is room for God's grace and mercy in all this.

But what you can do is choose fruits over pastries. You can choose water over coke. You can choose grilled chicken over fried chicken. You can choose healthier whole-grain breads over white breads. You can choose nuts and seeds over cookies. You can make sure you eat the 'herbs of the field' as you are commanded to do. You can choose mahi-mahi over catfish. You can choose steak over lobster. And in all cases, you can choose to not overeat. Start with what you can control. Be faithful in those things that you can control. This obedience to God's dietary directives will certainly enable you to experience good health and enable you to reach your ideal body weight.

Regardless of the specifics of the struggles you might face in the 'real world,' turn to God's Word, prayer, and worship to lead you to the right thing to do and the strength to follow through. God is anxious to partner with those who seek to please Him with a pure heart. God will honor your earnest commitment with blessings.

"Who shall ascend into the hill of the Lord*? or who shall stand in his holy place? He that hath clean hands, and a pure heart; who hath not lifted up his soul unto vanity, nor sworn deceitfully. He shall receive the blessing from the* Lord*, and righteousness from the God of his salvation." (Psalm 24:3-5, KJV)*

"Blessed are the pure in heart: for they shall see God." (Matthew 5:8, KJV)
"It is of the Lord*'s mercies that we are not consumed, because his compassions fail not. They are new every morning: great is thy faithfulness." (Lamentations 3:22-24, KJV)*

The following reminders and personal commitments may help you as you seek to live out dietary holiness in the 'real world.'

I acknowledge and accept that eating the healthy foods God created for me is His will for my life.

I acknowledge that God's plans for me are good, and that His blessings can only come to fruition to the extent that I follow His directives for my life.

I acknowledge that God has communicated to me the substances that are 'to be my food.'

I understand that Satan seeks to destroy me, as well as my loved ones; spiritually, emotionally, physically, and even eternally.

I can see that Satan has counterfeited God's dietary plan for me. I refuse to be a co-conspirator with Satan to destroy my body, sidetrack me from God's good plans for my life, cripple the Body of Christ, and hurt those that I love and am called to serve.

The way I conduct myself in accordance with God's Word during this life will affect me and others positively now, and in the life to come.

You will fail at times. I fail personally, and I fail to successfully lead my family at times. But then we fail in every area of our lives. Just because you gossiped today doesn't mean you can't repent and get back on the right path tomorrow. You will need to do the same thing with respect to your obedience to dietary holiness as well. But by working together, first recognizing that dietary holiness applies to us today, we can work to fail less often. That is why it is so important to spark a dietary reformation in the Church, so we can openly support and encourage one another.

It is important that you understand that, much like the recovering alcoholic, obedience to dietary holiness will require a daily commitment and involve a daily battle. For those of us who have struggled with our diets and the treatment of our bodies, we can never assume that we've 'got this.' If we are not spiritually prepared and ready each and every day, we may find ourselves flat on our backs in defeat before we even know what hit us.

Just as with any area of addiction that has once controlled our lives, a daily commitment and devotion to God's will for your life with regard to dietary holiness will be essential. We are all born with a sin nature that tends to have a bent towards certain areas of sin, while having no struggle in other areas. Some Believers have sin natures that have a bent towards gambling, sex, homosexuality, materialism, or power and control, while having no issue with food and junk non-foods, aside from not knowing that God wants them to eat healthy.

If you are reading this book it might be fair to assume that you, like me, have a bent towards unhealthy eating. Maybe like the AA alcoholic who always designates himself as a 'recovering alcoholic,' even after completing 1000 days without alcohol, you and I will need to always see ourselves as 'recovering eat-a-holics' who must look to God and His Word each day for strength to overcome the tendencies/bent of our sin natures.

By the way, don't spend a lot of time trying to determine why you are drawn to one area of sin or another. Don't try to determine if it was how your father treated you or if some series of events brought certain desires into your life. It really doesn't matter, with the exception of a possible need to forgive someone for how they treated you. You may have what might be considered valid reasons for being driven to some fleshly outlet, but in the end, you must give your body over to God. It is not yours to destroy, regardless of the source of the motivation.

There is no point in wasting your time, energy, and money trying to get to the bottom of it all, because ultimately, at the bottom of it all is where you will still be. It is enough to know which areas of sin you are drawn to, and to combat each with the wisdom and power of God available to you.

I know what I am talking about. I have a 4" thick file entitled Self-Analysis. It includes everything in there from personality and career tests to mini-documentaries of what makes Scott Lowery tick. I never profited one iota from all the self-analysis that I performed over the course of about 40 years of my life. As a matter of fact, it kept me from seeking God, rather relying on what man might devise to give me the breakthrough in my life that I so desperately needed.

"A fool hath no delight in understanding, but that his heart may discover itself." (Proverbs 18:2, KJV)

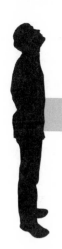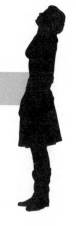

Chapter 26

Anorexia & Bulimia

For most of you, reaching your ideal body weight will mean that your body weight will decrease. But then there are some of you for whom reaching your ideal body weight will mean that your body weight will actually need to increase.

The principles of dietary holiness apply equally to everyone, for those who are overweight, for those who are underweight, and for everyone in between. Whether we are overweight, underweight, or just right, every Believer is called to walk out their lives in obedience to God's dietary directives.

I recently spoke with a young lady who had suffered with anorexic behavior at one point in her life. I will refer to her by the name of Stacy. Stacy had allowed her body weight to reach as low as 95 pounds, some 35 pounds below her ideal body weight. At her lowest weight, Stacy tried on a pair of size 0 shorts. She was so small that they slide right down her hips and legs to the ground.

Stacy would count calories and fat grams as closely as possible, seeking to stay at or below 1000 calories per day. And she would weigh herself regularly to make sure she did not gain any weight. Looking in the mirror, Stacy always saw someone who needed to lose more weight. As small as she was, lacking in any healthy level of musculature on her deprived body, she was always cold. Stacy would sometimes turn the oven on and stand or sit nearby to keep warm.

Although Stacy would never touch candies and pastries herself, she liked to feed those things to her husband and to others. She took pride in knowing that she could resist the desire to eat those things while others could not. She also liked the idea of others gaining weight so that her body weight and size would appear ever-smaller by comparison.

I am not going to try to determine the psychological and emotional path that someone must travel down to find themselves in the grip of anorexic and/or bulimic addiction. In a way, it really doesn't matter. What matters is that each of us, including those suffering from anorexic and bulimic tendencies, understand and obey God's Word regarding diet and health. In the process of walking in obedience to God's Word concerning diet and health I believe that those psychological and emotional issues will be resolved.

I addressed this earlier, but it is worth repeating here. Don't spend a lot of time trying to determine why you are drawn to one area of sin or another. And make no mistake about it, anorexic and bulimic behaviors are sinful behaviors.

Don't try to determine if it was how your father treated you or if some series of events brought certain desires into your life. It really doesn't matter, with the exception of a possible need to forgive someone for how they treated you. You may have what might be considered valid reasons for being driven to some fleshly outlet, but in the end, you must give your body over to God. It is not yours to destroy, regardless of the source of the motivation.

There is no point in wasting your time, energy, and money trying to get to the bottom of it all, because ultimately, at the bottom of it all is where you will still be. It is enough to know which areas of sin you are drawn to, and to combat each with the wisdom and power of God available to you.

I know what I am talking about. I have a 4" thick file entitled Self-Analysis. It includes everything in there from personality and career tests to mini-documentaries of what makes Scott Lowery tick. I never profited one iota from all the self-analysis that I performed over the course of about 40 years of my life. As a matter of fact, it kept me from seeking God; rather relying on what man might devise to give me the breakthrough in my life that I so desperately needed.

"A fool hath no delight in understanding, but that his heart may discover itself." (Proverbs 18:2, KJV)

All the principles of dietary holiness found in this book apply equally to those who suffer from gluttony, to those who suffer from anorexia or bulimia, and to those who suffer from neither. At the expense of being redundant, it might be helpful for those suffering with anorexia or bulimia to get a review of these principles of dietary holiness, maybe pointed a bit more in their direction.

Exercise is not necessary to reach your ideal body weight. If you are suffering from anorexic or bulimic tendencies, you may be guilty of excessive exercise. Most especially for you, moving away from a focused exercise program will be an important first step. For many, a focused exercise program is actually a form of bulimia. Trust that living out your life in a Godly manner will give you all of the physical activity that you need, while keeping your focus off your body.

There are five spiritual keys to reaching your ideal body weight. First, you must acknowledge that your body is not your own, but that it is under God's ownership. You must recognize that anorexic and bulimic behaviors represent poor management of God's property. Your view of your body and what you think and want it to look like are of no consequence. You are to obey God's directives regarding diet and health and to trust Him to work His will and way in your life and in your body.

Second, spiritual conditioning is a prerequisite to physical conditioning. You must dedicate time daily to the study of God's Word, prayer, and worship in order to overcome your fleshly tendencies towards anorexia or bulimia.

Third, listen to the guidance of the Holy Spirits leading in your life. If you are experiencing shame for your anorexic and/or bulimic behaviors, take pause and consider what the Holy Spirit is trying to say to you.

Fourth, pursue purposeful living. Whatever pleasure you have deceived yourself into believing can only be achieved by living at a low body weight, and by the pride of believing that you can control what you eat while others cannot, will never satisfy. The pursuit of pleasure in life will never lead to a life of purpose. It's within the context of a purpose-filled life that your draw to such destructive pleasures will dissipate.

And five, a righteous motivation is required to reach your ideal body weight. If pride is at the root of your motivation in life, your motivation for controlling your diet, then reaching your ideal body weight will be extremely difficult. Pride will always go before a fall, before failure.

Adhere to God's basic diet plan as outlined in Ecclesiastes 10:17. Eat in due season – Eat when your body is calling for food. This is very important for those suffering from anorexic and bulimic tendencies. Eat for strength – Eat God's healthy foods not man's junk non-foods. Eat not for drunkenness – Don't use eating as an escape. This point might apply more to those suffering from bulimia than to those suffering from anorexia.

Consider the seven practical suggestions for reaching your ideal body weight. In summary, include the following items in your diet each day ...

1) One to two tablespoons of cod-liver oil or flaxseed oil (Omega-3 source)
2) One piece of fruit and one salad (life-force and fiber)
3) Two pieces of Ezekiel 4:9 bread (reduced carb cravings)
4) Eat eggs several times each week, if not daily (nutrient-dense)

5) Eat dark green leafy vegetables several times each week, if not daily (nutrient-dense)

6) Eliminate caffeine (removal of chemically-induced stress and nutrient drain)

7) Keep a bottle of water with you at all times (detoxification process)

Implementing these suggestions alone will quickly begin moving you from your anorexic body weight to your ideal body weight, providing your body with the nutrients of which it has been deprived.

Carefully consider what stresses in your life need to be handled or eliminated through God's wisdom and direction. Have you placed yourself in environments that have worked to tear you down spiritually and emotionally? You may need to make some changes in how you do life.

What you eat matters to God. Your diet matters to God. He is concerned over your anorexic and/or bulimic tendencies. God wants you free from this life of addiction that controls you and damages your body. Don't allow man's misinterpretation of Scripture to convince you otherwise.

Remember that you are called to be a witness to the world, to live above all the nations, and to glorify God in your body. An underweight and malnourished body fails to accomplish this God-ordained calling in your life

Don't weigh yourself and avoid looking at yourself in the mirror as much as possible. And don't measure yourself either. Don't give your flesh any opportunity to get involved. Eat as God directs and trust Him for the right results. And don't count calories and fat grams. For all of us, that has got to be the silliest waste of time man has ever devised.

God does not want any of us to become health nuts, to become obsessed with our bodies. But what He does want is for you to obey His dietary directives and trust Him for the right results in your life and in your body. It is birthright to live out your life at your ideal body weight. This is God's will for your life. Walk in it.

In Conclusion

In the Introduction chapter of this book I suggested that when trying to discern what is the truth of Scripture regarding diet and health, or any other topic, you should apply the following acid test to differentiate between what is true and what is false.

1) Are the principles found in this book balanced with respect to God's love, God's holiness, and God's sovereignty? Have you not found that dietary holiness strikes the perfect balance? God desires to love us through dietary holiness. The holiness of God, the holy life He calls us to, and the witness we are to be to the world, is exemplified in dietary holiness. God is sovereign in that our bodies are His to control through His dietary directives. Our bodies are no longer our own.

2) When deciding between two opposite Biblical views, break the tie by determining which view gives God the most glory. Have you not found that dietary holiness, as opposed to dietary deception, will give God the most glory? A healthy, fit, and long-living Church has the potential to draw more people to God (glorify God) than any evangelical movement in history.

3) The Bible says we will know evil by its evil fruit. Determine which view leads towards righteous fruit and which view leads towards evil fruit. Have you not found that dietary holiness produces righteous fruit and that dietary deception produces evil fruit? Dietary deception has produced a Church that is tired, sick, overweight, and living a fraction of the years God intended (evil fruit). It will be dietary

holiness that works to produce a Church that is the most healthy demographic on the planet (good fruit).

God wants you delivered from fatigue, sickness, excess weight, and all of the emotional struggles that come with it. God has called you to be a positive witness to the world of the wisdom and power of His ways. He has given you His word to guide you in the truth necessary to accomplish these things in your life.

I know that you do not want to pass down a heritage of spiritual, emotional, and physical weakness to your children and grandchildren. You do not want them to suffer as you have. You have determined that you are willing to go against the grain of society, to no longer live life by the patterns of this world.

For the Believer, you now realize that your body was purchased by God when you accepted Jesus Christ as your Savior. Your body is no longer your own. You are commanded to glorify God in your body.

You have seen that God does care greatly about what you eat, your health, and your body weight. You have seen that God has provided you with instruction and directives in that regard. And you have seen that nothing that Jesus could have possibly done on the cross would have changed God's concern for your diet and health, or His requirement for holy living towards His people, Old and New Testament Church alike.

You have seen that spiritual conditioning, acknowledging that your body is not your own, living a purpose-driven life, listening closely to the voice of the Holy Spirit, and a righteous motivation are the keys to give you the strength to follow through with dietary holiness in your life. And you have learned that there is a physical-emotional-spiritual connection that comes into play in an important way.

You have seen the evidence that God's people have been living apart from God's dietary directives, both in the poor quality of life lived out and the reduced quantity of life that God intended for His people. You have seen that God's people must live a sober life to change this.

You have learned that God's Word has the answers to all of life's tough questions and struggles, to include relative to your health and body weight. And that God's wisdom, not man's wisdom, is where you need to go to find out what it takes to achieve success in your life.

We have 'rightly divided the word of truth' to reveal numerous Scriptures that have been misinterpreted, even modified, to support dietary deception in the Church. Through it all you have been able to see that the perversion of God's created foods into refined sugars, for example, and its consumption, constitutes sin in your life.

You have learned that the Church should be the healthiest demographic on the planet, a beacon of hope, Biblical wisdom, and successful living to a world that looks on in search of the 'Real Thing' for their own lives.

The tendency of our flesh with regard to the truths of Scripture regarding diet is to scream, 'But that's too hard! It can't be true if it's that hard!' But we are, in fact, as Believers, called to keep ourselves unspotted from the world around us, whether in how we approach our marriages, how we approach our work, how we approach our finances, or how we approach our diets.

"Pure religion and undefiled before God and the Father is this, to visit the fatherless and widows in their affliction, and to keep himself unspotted from the world." (James 1:27, KJV)

What is harder, loving your spouse when they have been unkind to you or choosing an orange over a donut? Loving your spouse. But no one would ever argue that this standard of holy living regarding marriage can't be true because it is too hard.

What is harder, not gossiping or choosing grilled chicken over fried chicken? Not gossiping. But no one would ever argue that this standard of holy living regarding gossip can't be true because it is too hard.

You get the idea. It only 'seems' harder than every other requirement of holy living because we have never acknowledged that such a call of God on our lives even exists (the ultimate secret sin). Add to this that the Church won't support dietary holiness and won't support you in upholding it, you find yourself on your own. I suppose in this way it could be argued that dietary holiness is harder than other areas of holy living.

At least with other areas of holy living you can seek council and support from the Church more readily. At least with other areas of holy living you can expect to be encouraged from the pulpit to walk in obedience. You are not likely to get that from the pulpit concerning dietary holiness. But you can be a part of changing all that by reaching your ideal body weight God's Weigh.

I am hopeful for you. My hope is not a wish. My hope for you is founded in the promises, wisdom, and power of God's Word. I know that the same promises, wisdom, and power that have set me free from addiction to food, unhealthy eating, and poor health will do the same for you.

Working together in truth through Christ Jesus, we can overturn the dietary deception of Satan that has worked to destroy God's people spiritually, emotionally, and physically. The Christian Community will move from deception, bondage, weakness, and pain to enlightenment, freedom, strength, and peace.

We should be thankful to God for His patience and longsuffering concerning our dietary disobedience. Although the consequences have certainly been severe enough, they could be so much worse. It amazes me that our bodies can take the abuse we subject them to for more than a year or two, much less seventy to eighty years. Our sinfulness in this regard warrants a much more swift reward, but that is not God's way.

"He hath not dealt with us after our sins; nor rewarded us according to our iniquities." (Psalm 103:10, KJV)

God still desires to show you the truth, to give you another chance.

He wants you to see the wisdom and power of His ways in your life. He wants you to see that His precepts will deliver you from fatigue, sickness, excess weight, and emotional pain.

God created all things. He created your body. God created and designated those substances that are to be food for your body. And He created these foods in the form necessary to nourish your body. We are not to tamper with His design.

God is your source for all wisdom concerning all things, certainly to include diet and health. It pleases God when you make Him your sole source. You may have spent many years and decades seeking truth from mankind, and quite frankly, the devices of Satan. You may have lived far away from the ways of God concerning diet and health. But you are now ready to turn away from your dietary sins unto dietary holiness. This is a great moment in your spiritual journey.

We have all alienated ourselves from God's truths at times. We have become enemies of the way and will of God in our lives. But you are ready to come home to God and His ways. Your prodigal journey is finally over. You are ready to let go and let God in your life, diet and body weight included. You are ready to reach your ideal body weight.

God's truth concerning diet and health may have seemed as a mystery to you. This is largely because the Church has refused to seek and acknowledge God's truth in this regard. Also, as motivated by our carnal natures, we have not only avoided the truth, but we have even worked to distort it. For you, God's truth concerning diet and health is a mystery no more.

I desire to speak the truth of God to you, warning every Believer of Satan's devices against us, teaching each of the wisdom and power of God's ways, so that we may present ourselves whole in Christ Jesus, thoroughly furnished unto all good works. Relative to diet and health, the Christian community has been spoiled through the traditions and wisdom of man, living after the patterns of this world, and not living after the wisdom and ways of God.

You will never be free from bondage to unhealthy eating and excess weight until you recognize that you can only be complete, not lacking in any good thing, when you turn to God for the solution to your struggles, failures, and concerns. Now is your time to do that. Now is your time to reach your ideal body weight.

You are called to deny your fleshly lusts and the sins of your flesh. You are called to make all your decisions in favor of the working of God and His truths in your life. You are called to be wise and to overcome the deceptions of Satan in your life. You are called to live life at your ideal body weight.

For those who would insist that dietary holiness does not apply to them, I would encourage them to carefully consider their spiritual condition. They should ask themselves the question 'If it were true, would I obey anyway?' Are they holding onto something they wouldn't give over to God anyway? They should ask themselves 'Can I handle the truth?'

"… he that hath ears to hear, let him hear." (Luke 8:8, KJV)

"For every one that doeth evil hateth the light, neither cometh to the light, lest his deeds should be reproved." (John 3:20, KJV)

"And these are they which are sown among thorns; such as hear the word, And the cares of this world, and the deceitfulness of riches, and the lusts of other things entering in, choke the word, and it becometh unfruitful." (Mark 4:18-19, KJV)

The unwillingness of some to accept the words in this book as truth may be based on their belief that nobody else is doing it and most people will think this is crazy. I would submit to them, as I have studied through the Bible over the past several decades, that the Biblical pattern played out over and over again is that 'the majority is never right.' The way to truth, for those willing to find it, is often down a very narrow path, seldom the wide commonly traveled path.

"Many will follow their shameful ways and will bring the way of truth into disrepute." (II Peter 2:2, KJV)

Some might contend that the principles in this book cannot be true because they have not been presented in this way before now. Why now? How can it be that a book like this has not been written before? What Biblical insights could Scott Lowery possibly have that it seems no one else in the Church has had before?

I can only offer a guess or opinion as to why a presentation of dietary holiness as found in this book has not been made before, at least not to this extent. I know it is not because God has wanted to 'hide' the truth from anyone. But I wonder if God sometimes allows certain things to 'wait in the wings' for a significantly noticeable release that can have a major impact in the lives of His people and around the world, as opposed to a simmering truth that slowly grows and develops over time. Like Esther, were I and this book created for such a time as this?

I think about Noah's ark as an example of this possibility. It seems highly unlikely that our ability to find and obtain clear photos of Noah's ark would be by accident. It seems that God has done a really good job of keeping Noah's ark from being found and photographed. With all our modern technology, God has managed to keep it hidden. Even the Titanic was located some 2 1/2 miles beneath the ocean's surface.

I cannot help but to wonder if God is waiting to allow the clear location and photography of Noah's ark to occur at a time that will have the greatest evangelical impact possible. Just imagine the witness to the world that finding and photographing Noah's ark will be. It would be an incredible testimony of the truth and accuracy of the Bible to a doubting world.

For those who have heard, received, and will apply the truth of dietary holiness to their own lives, I would encourage you to work to take it another step further. We need to work to get the entire Church on board. We can do this in a number of ways.

1) The Church must realize that there is such a thing as dietary holiness, and that it applies to Believers today.

2) The Church must quit picking and choosing what it wants and doesn't want from the Old Testament.

3) The Church needs to take this issue seriously, no longer joking amongst its members and from the pulpit.

4) The Church must quit pushing the drug of junk non-foods on its members and their children.

5) The Church leadership must begin to rally against dietary deception with the type of focus and programs they have provided regarding every other category of holy living.

6) The Church must work together to support and disciple one another in the area of dietary holiness.

7) The Church must focus on accountability through transparency and encouragement.

Dietary holiness has the power to bring on a whole new era in the Church, a witness to the world that may lead more people to Christ than any movement in history. It all starts with your obedience to God's dietary directives and achieving health and an ideal body weight in your own life. Please help to lead the charge towards a dietary reformation in the Church.

"And the very God of peace sanctify you wholly; and I pray God your whole spirit and soul and body be preserved blameless unto the coming of our Lord Jesus Christ." (I Thessalonians 5:23, KJV)

Look to God and His Word for all truth. Never inherit your theology from man.

"For as the heavens are higher than the earth, so are my ways higher than your ways, and my thoughts than your thoughts." (Isaiah 55:9, KJV)

"My son, attend to my words; incline thine ear unto my sayings. Let them not depart from thine eyes; keep them in the midst of thine heart. For they are life unto those that find them, and health to all their flesh." (Proverbs 4:20-22, KJV)

You have the truth regarding dietary holiness and you know how to develop the spiritual strength necessary to follow through with it in obedience. There is now nothing standing between you and your ideal body weight. You now know God's Weigh to Your Ideal Body Weight.

A Final Plea

The Church is tired, sick, overweight, and living a fraction of the years God intended. This is not God's will for His people. Where have we gone wrong? Have we not simply followed the dietary pattern of this world?

Contrary to popular opinion, a variety of common misconceptions, and numerous Biblical misinterpretations (dietary deception), God's principles concerning diet and health are not suggestions to be considered, but rather, are commandments to be obeyed.

God's Word speaks very clearly to what we should eat, how much we should eat, when we should eat, and why we should eat. In Biblical principle, it even speaks to the perversions of God's created and prescribed foods: refined sugars, refined flours, and hydrogenated oils, for example. And God's Word shows us how to wage spiritual warfare to overcome our inability to control our diets, which at its core, is a spiritual issue.

Dietary deception is tearing away at the spiritual, emotional, and physical health of God's people and the witness to the world we are called to be.

Just picture a healthy Church. The world would be beating down our church doors to find out what we were doing differently, why we were doing it differently, and most importantly, Who told us to do it differently. In this way, obedience to God's Word concerning diet and health could be one of the greatest evangelical tools the Church has ever known.

If we do not change our dietary ways, what heritage will we leave for our children? It will be one of fatigue, diabetes, cardiovascular disease, cancer, arthritis, excess weight, and emotional instability. We are already seeing that. And even more importantly, we will leave our children without the spiritual training and strength necessary to control their fleshly desires.

We are raising our children to be the next generation of the tired, sick, and overweight Church, with lifespans even shorter than ours. They deserve better from their parents and Sunday-School teachers. Despite the best of intentions, this is not the loving thing to do.

The Church has been guilty of watering down the definition, application, and power of God's grace. Grace is meant to overcome evil, not allow it. Shall we continue in sin that grace may abound? God forbid.

Sin is any perversion of, or deviation from, God's plan, purpose, or design. Sin leads to pain, harm, enslavement, and shame. God's Word clearly communicates that we will know evil by its evil fruit. And for the Believer, our bodies are no longer our own, to be destroyed by our fleshly lusts.

No matter how you slice it, an unhealthy diet is a sinful diet. It is just that simple. God's ways are always simple, effective, never-changing, and freeing. It will be Satan's ways that are complicated, ineffective, ever-changing, and enslaving. By which 'way' have we become tired, sick, and overweight? It most certainly hasn't been God's Weigh.

The Church must acknowledge its unhealthy dietary practices as sin. If we refuse, we will remain tired, sick, and overweight, living the years allotted a sinful people. We will limp along in spiritual and emotional bondage, a mere shadow of what God has called us to be.

God is calling for a dietary reformation in the Church. Won't you answer His call?

The Purpose for This Book and God's Weigh Ministry

Through this book and God's Weigh Ministry I seek to minister to the Body of Christ and to you personally. I have a vision, a mission, and set of values that govern and direct this ministry effort.

I envision a Body of Christ that experiences the vibrant physical health and ideal body weight for each member that God has always intended and desired for His people. God's people should be so statistically healthier than the rest of the world, and live so significantly longer, that the world would be drawn to the One who has blessed our temporal bodies through His Word, and more importantly, the One who can save their eternal souls.

The mission of this book and ministry is to show the Body of Christ that following God's Word concerning diet and health is about walking in obedience, our reasonable service. The mission of this book and ministry is to enlighten the Body of Christ to the reality that the issue of diet affects our entire being; spiritually, emotionally, and physically.

The mission of this book and ministry is to educate the Body of Christ relative to the principles for experiencing physical health as God has outlined in His Word, by working to facilitate the dietary reformation so needed within the Church. The mission of this book and ministry is to expose the deceptions of Satan that have laid the foundation for the decline in physical health we are seeing within the Body of Christ. The mission of this book and ministry is to lead you to your ideal body weight.

The foundation of this book and ministry is based on a number of core values/beliefs. I believe that God's Word has the answers to all of life's questions, for the blessing of spirit, soul, and body. I believe that God's people should be the healthiest people on Earth. I believe that God's people should stand apart from the world in every facet of life, including physical health and body weight.

I believe it is foolish for any to believe that Jesus' work on the cross would free us to destroy our bodies by enslaving us to the god of food and an unhealthy diet. I believe that a loving God would never give permission to His children to harm themselves by destroying their physical bodies with the dietary perversions of Satan, as well as spiritually and emotionally in the process. I believe that to believe otherwise constitutes Biblical heresy, which I believe is exactly the manner by which the Church is presently operating concerning diet and health.

I believe that the proper care of your body is your reasonable service to God, Who has purchased your body for a price through the life, death, and resurrection of His Son, Jesus Christ. God has not suggested that you be a good steward of your body. God has purchased the right to, and has in fact, commanded that you be a good steward of your body.

I believe that true transformation in any area of life is a direct by-product of spiritual growth. God's people are not suffering from a lack of dietary knowledge, but rather, God's people are lacking the spiritual enlightenment and strength necessary to walk in obedience to God's Word, preferring to reside in a place of spiritual darkness, that they might maintain their secret sin and continue in the lusts of their flesh.

I believe that Satan has been tremendously effective in keeping God's people from the blessing of physical health and their ideal body weight, and the resulting witness to the world it could be. I believe it is time to change that through the accurate interpretation and application of God's Word to our lives. I believe that the Bible is the greatest health and weight loss book ever written.

I believe God wants you to achieve and live out your life at your ideal body weight. I believe this is the birthright of every Believer.

If the Body of Christ is tired, sick, and overweight, it is our own fault.

We have failed to seek God's wisdom. We have refused to deny the lusts of our flesh. We have conformed to the pattern of this world. Will we now repent and turn to God?

God has equipped me with an insatiable desire to understand His Word and find practical application to everyday life. I desire to work to help perfect and edify the Body of Christ towards His more perfect will for each of our lives. Concerning diet and health, the study and pursuit of dietary holiness represents a significant effort and achievement in that regard.

God has created me to be a reformer, a teacher, and a writer. It is my pleasure to serve God and my fellow man through this book; to be in the business of perfecting the saints, and edifying the Body of Christ, for the work of the ministry. It is my pleasure to help you reach your ideal body weight through the practical application of God's Word.

"And He gave some, apostles; and some, prophets; and some, evangelists; and some, pastors and teachers; For the perfecting of the saints, for the work of the ministry, for the edifying of the body of Christ: Till we all come in the unity of the faith, and of the knowledge of the Son of God, unto a perfect man, unto the measure of the stature of the fullness of Christ: That we henceforth be no more children, tossed to and fro, carried about with every wind of doctrine, by the sleight of men, and cunning craftiness whereby they lie in wait to deceive; But speaking the truth in love, may grow up into Him in all things, which is the head, even Christ." (Ephesians 4:11-15, KJV)

The reason I believe God has called me to write this book is because our dietary practices represent an area of required obedience in which the Church is the absolute furthest from God's wisdom and ways. Unhealthy eating has become the Church's 'drug of choice,' and like most addicts, we don't want to talk about it. We are suffering tremendously in spirit, soul, and body from this problem. We are clearly in need of a dietary reformation in the Church.

Most of God's people deny that God's dietary plan even applies to the New Testament Church to begin with. We prefer to believe that the work of Jesus on the cross somehow delivered us from any need or requirement to be good stewards of our bodies. Despite popular opinion, various common misconceptions, and numerous Biblical misinterpretations, the Bible does address God's directives and expectations for our lives with regard to diet and health.

Please allow the reading of this book to equip you with the same vision, mission, values, and concern. Allow this book to lead you to the physical health and ideal body weight that God desires for you.

Working together in Biblical truth through Christ Jesus, we can overturn the dietary deceptions of Satan that have worked to destroy God's people spiritually, emotionally, and physically. The Christian community can move from deception, bondage, weakness, and pain to enlightenment, freedom, strength, and peace. And you will reach your ideal body weight in the process.

What's Next for God's Weigh Ministry & What You Can Do to Help

I will continue to work with the Church, through this ministry and this book, to spark the dietary reformation so needed. I will do this through the marketing of this book, my website, seminars, book-signings, television and radio broadcasts, social media, and any other venue to which God might lead me.

But I need your help. God will call upon an army of Believers to both lead His people to dietary holiness and to be a witness to the world of the wisdom and power of God. First and foremost, you must begin to walk out dietary holiness in your own life. And then, you should begin to work to minister to others in the same way you have been blessed through this book/ministry and dietary holiness.

You can reach out to others by pointing them to God's wisdom concerning diet and health, by directing them to this book and ministry, by setting an example of dietary holiness, and by encouraging your church leadership to address the matter of dietary holiness in their lives and with respect to their congregation. You can begin support groups and study groups within your church to support dietary holiness in each of your lives.

God's Weigh to Your Ideal Body Weight is all about reaching your ideal body weight through the wisdom and power of God as it concerns our basic dietary choices. But there is so much more work to be done.

My next book, *God's Weigh in a Real World*, will take matters to a whole new level. In addition to expanding upon the principles found in this book and other components of the Biblical Doctrine of Physical Health, *God's Weigh in a Real World* will work to develop a plan that the Church can use to take on the medical establishment, the junk non-food industry, pharmaceutical companies, the government school system, the government, and even the fitness industry regarding the need for a dietary reformation in this country; reformation in all things fitness really. I am not trying to contend that these systems are not full of good, well-meaning people, but that these systems, as a whole, are broken regarding the Biblical Doctrine of Physical Health.

Through our voices, our votes, and our purchasing power, we can get these establishments moving in the right direction, regardless of how unwilling they may be. We can let them know what we will and will not stand for. Relative to our purchasing power, rest assured that these establishments will work to reposition themselves in the direction the Church spends its money. For example, buy more of God's foods and they will provide more of God's foods. Buy more organic foods and they will provide more organic foods, and more cheaply.

Please don't be impatient for this next book. We have plenty to do over the next several years just getting the Church on board with what this book addresses, dietary holiness. But I did want to give you a glimpse of things to come, Lord willing. In the meantime, we must first get the plank out of our own eye. I hope and pray that you will join me in this worthy fight.